Ureteral Complications of Gynecological Surgery

Jean-Bernard Dubuisson
Jean Dubuisson · Martina Martins Favre
Gregory J. Wirth

Ureteral Complications of Gynecological Surgery

Prevention, Diagnosis and Treatment

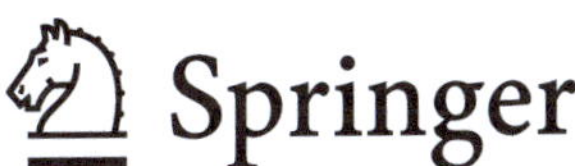
Springer

Jean-Bernard Dubuisson
Gynecology Department
Institut Médico-Chirurgical De Champel
Geneva, Switzerland

Martina Martins Favre
Radiology Department
Imagerive Center
Geneva, Switzerland

Jean Dubuisson
Gynecological Surgery Unit
Geneva University Hospitals and
University of Geneva
Geneva, Switzerland

Gregory J. Wirth
Urology Department
University Hospitals of Geneva
Geneva, Switzerland

ISBN 978-3-031-15600-7   ISBN 978-3-031-15598-7   (eBook)
https://doi.org/10.1007/978-3-031-15598-7

This Springer imprint is published by the registered company Springer Nature Switzerland AG
The registered company address is: Gewerbestrasse 11, 6330 Cham, Switzerland

Acknowledgments

My true affection to my family, Catherine my wife, Pierre, Paul, and Jean our sons who have supported and encouraged me in my endeavors for many years. A special thought to Jean who followed me on the long difficult trip of gynecological surgery. He dominates perfectly all facets of gynecological surgery. A deep gratitude to Dr. Martina Martins Favre, eminent radiologist, who contributed to this book with her special knowledge of urology imaging. My thanks go to Dr. Greggory Wirth, urologist and well-known surgeon who wrote the chapter concerning the surgery of the ureter. He managed to do it in the hands of a master.

J. B. Dubuisson

Contents

Why This Book?

1

J.-B. Dubuisson et al., *Ureteral Complications of Gynecological Surgery*,
https://doi.org/10.1007/978-3-031-15598-7_1

This book is a practical reference book for gynecologists and surgeons. It includes all the questions and answers that one can ask about the ureter in gynecology.

## 1.1	As a Pelvic Surgeon, Knowledge About the Ureter Should Be Important

Even after learning, we do not know sufficiently…, especially in surgery. This book is made for helping all abdominal and pelvic surgeons.

This book is written specially for gynecologists and pelvic surgeons. We started from the idea that gynecologists and surgeons need an easy practical reference book including all the questions and answers that one can ask about the ureter in gynecology. We think it is important for a gynecologist surgeon to have a book of reference containing most of the knowledge needed in gynecology concerning the ureter. It is the reason why the chapters are varied, and concern anatomy, histology, laparoscopic evaluations, prevention and description of injuries of the ureter, including imagery and management of the complications.

## 1.2	The Ureter, Taboo for Gynecologists?

The ureter, in gynecology, is rather a taboo subject that we, gynecologists, avoid talking about it. If we talk about it, usually it is for a perioperative complication that should be solved quickly, to avoid more severe problems.

## 1.3	The Ureter, the Main Organ in Pelvic Surgery

Whatever these considerations, the ureter is an important topic of work in gynecological surgery. When a ureteral lesion is suspected during surgery, an accurate assessment should be made immediately. If there is any doubt of injury of the ureter, additional surgical procedures are to be discussed: evaluation, ureterolysis, cystoscopy, and intravenous indigo carmine injection, JJ stent placement. Also, if there are any unexpected urinary symptoms in the postoperative course, a complete evaluation must be established, especially with imaging, as soon as possible. To miss a urinary complication is always dramatic.

## 1.4	The Ureter, a Calm Neighbor

The ureter has always been a close and calm neighbor for gynecological and pelvic surgeons. Its proximity explains why gynecologists have been interested in it for a long time. The ureter is solitary, not intrusive, and autonomous. Even sometimes, it is of great help when it alarms because of its presence next to abnormal gynecological lesions by its pain or renal colic. On the other hand, sometimes, our problem is that "we injure the ureter" during gynecological surgery, but always unintentionally and accidentally.

## 1.5	The Ureter and Litigation

The ureter, accidentally injured, is the main cause of litigation in gynecological surgery. That is the reason why established and experimented surgeons respect it unanimously. This explains why the young surgeons fear being too close.

## 1.6	Constant Vision of the Ureter During Pelvic Surgery

Every time we perform a laparotomy, a laparoscopy, or a vaginal access surgery for pelvic pathology, we look at it. The good and experienced surgeon always sees, locates, and inspects it quickly. It will be felt with the finger or with atraumatic forceps. Stressed surgeons are always worried when they navigate around.

Before, several years ago, surgeons who had not seen it said to themselves: "not seen, not taken." Today, this joke is no longer valid. Ghozzi rightly writes in these terms: "You have to see the ureter and avoid it, rather than avoiding seeing it" [1].

1.7 Ureter Frowned upon or too Close to a Dissection Means Sometimes Stress for the Gynecologic Surgeon

Even experienced surgeons are sometimes worried about having operated too close to the ureter, with extensive electrocoagulation, with too much destruction of the surrounding tissue. Indeed, in these cases, there is a risk that it has been burnt by thermal diffusion. But it is very difficult to know immediately if the ureter was hit by a burn. We will know the verdict only after a few days. The novice surgeons are also attentive in case of surgical difficulties near the ureter. Then, simple intraoperative procedures should be made to control it. These procedures will be described in one of the chapters. It is certainly not necessary to wait until the injury gives symptoms. Surgeons must be proactive. A complication appearing in the postoperative course is a bigger problem to be diagnosed, and treat because of the overlying renal complications, that are always possible.

These are the main messages of this book.

Reference

1. Ghozzi S, Khiari R, Mlik K, Hmidi M, Ktari M, Khouni H, Hammami A, Fkih N, Hellel M, Ben RN. Les traumatismes de l'uretère d'origine gynécologique. Tunisie médicale. 2006;84(10):617–20.

Part I

Anatomy of the Ureter

Classic Anatomy 2

Chapter 2 includes everything we need to know about the general anatomy of the ureter for surgeons.

It seemed important to start this book with anatomical considerations, essential to know before any discussion on the place of the ureter in the gynecological surgery [1]. Classic anatomy is adapted to modern gynecological surgery [2].

2.1 General Anatomy (Fig. 2.1)

The ureter is the "active" tube that connects the kidney to the bladder. The ureters extend from the pyelon to the ureteral meatus in the bladder. The two ureters have a global direction downward and medially [1], 8 cm apart at their origin from each other, they are only 2 cm at their termination.

The diameter is approximately 10 mm in the lumbar segment, and 4 mm in the iliac and pelvic segments with two strictures, one at the level of the promontory, and the other at the entrance into the bladder wall. In the bladder wall, its diameter is 1–5 mm.

2.2 Dimensions of the Ureter (Fig. 2.2)

The dimensions of the ureter are roughly standard. Its length is 25 cm. The lumbar ureter is 6 cm, followed by the iliac ureter 3–4 cm. Then it measures 8–8.5 cm from the promontory to the crossing of the uterine artery. The ureter measures 3 cm from the crossing of the uterine artery to the wall of the bladder. Its intravesical intramural portion is 1.5 cm long. Its path in the bladder is oblique, submucous, and participates in the constitution of the trigone. The distance between the ureter and the uterine isthmus is 1.7 cm, between the ureter and the anterior vaginal cul-de-sac is 1.5–1.7 cm, and between the ureter and the lateral fornix is 1.2–1.3 cm.

The ureter is characteristic in its pale color, located in the retroperitoneal space, behind the peritoneum to which it adheres, having a mesentery with its vessels.

Fig. 2.1 General anatomy of the ureters. Right side. (1) Right kidney, (2) ureter, (3) iliac vessels, (4) light stenosis at the level of promontory, (5) light stenosis at the entrance in the bladder, (6) bladder

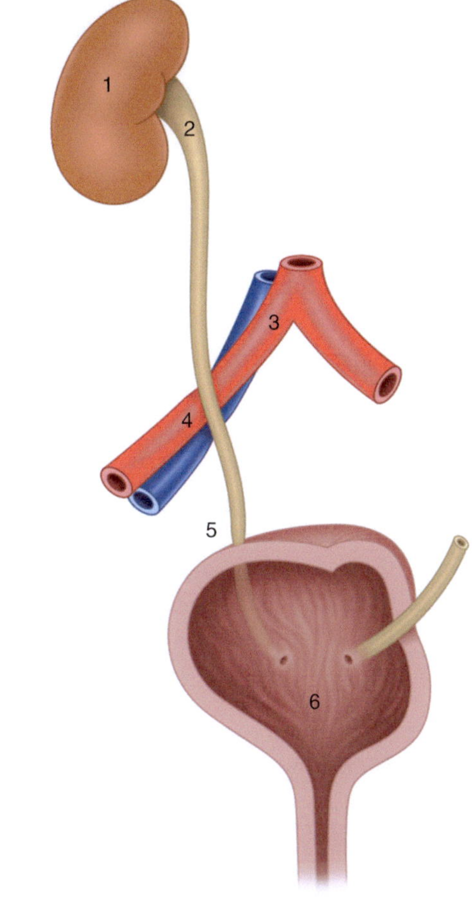

Fig. 2.2 Situation and dimensions of the ureters. (1) Left kidney, (2) left ovarian vein, (3) right renal vein, (4) left ureter, (5) right ureter, (6) vena cava, (7) right ovarian vein, (8) aorta, (9) bowel, (10) left ovary, (11) uterus, (12) right ovary, (13) left uterine artery, (14) inferior mesenteric artery

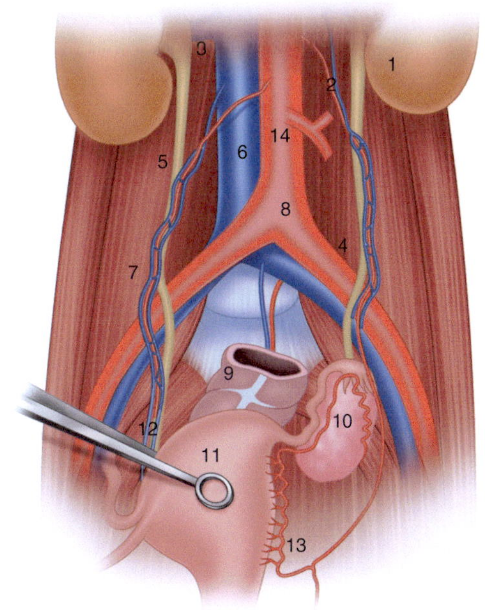

2.3 Anatomical Relationships of the Lumbar Segment (Fig. 2.3)

2.3.1 Dorsally

Dorsally, the relationships are the iliaca fascia and the psoas which separate it from the transverse processes of the lumbar spine.

2.3.2 Laterally

Laterally, we see the inner sub-hilar border of the kidney then the psoas bordered by the genitofemoral nerve (formerly called genitocrural), an important sensory nerve that innervates the genitals, especially the clitoris and the labia majora. Derived from the anterior roots of the first two lumbar nerves, it emerges from the psoas muscle and passes beneath the ureter from the midline to a lateral position.

2.3.3 Medially

Medially, the relationships are different on the right and left.

On the right, the ureter responds to the inferior vena cava and lymph nodes and, further away, to the lumbar sympathetic chain.

On the left, the ureter responds to the aorta.

2.3.4 Ventrally

Ventrally, the ratios are also different on the right and left.

On the right, the relationships of the ureter are the Treitz fascia (fascia of joining the dorsal sheet of the meso-duodenum with the dorsal parietal peritoneum) and the second duodenum. The line of attachment of the mesentery crosses it dorsally. The right colic and ileocolic arteries are related to the ventral aspect of the ureter.

On the left is found Todd's fascia, joining the left mesocolon with the left colic vessels which cross the ureter.

2.4 Crossing of the Infundibulopelvic Ligament (Fig. 2.2)

The ureters are crossed on both sides by the ovarian vessels, ventrally, in the area of the body of the fourth lumbar vertebra. The ovarian arteries arise from the aorta under the renal artery. But the left ovarian vein crosses the ureter higher than the right one, at the level of the third lumbar vertebra, flowing into the renal vein.

Fig. 2.3 Anatomical relationships of the lumbar segment. (1) Right kidney, (2) right adrenal gland, (3) inferior vena cava, (4) aorta, (5) celiac trunk, (6) pancreas, (7) splenic artery, (8) left adrenal gland, (9) left kidney, (10) duodenum, (11) ileal arteries, (12) jejunum, (13) psoas muscle and genitocrural nerve, (14) right ureter, (15) left ureter, (16) inferior mesenteric vein, (17) ovarian vessels

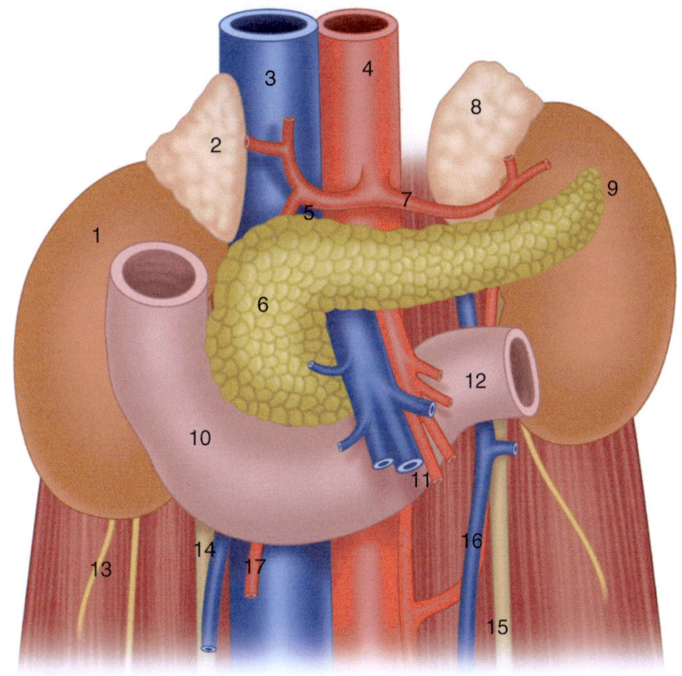

2.5 Anatomical Relationships of the Iliac Segment (Figs. 2.4, 2.5, 2.6 and 2.7)

2.5.1 Dorsally

Dorsally, the relationships of the iliac segment are the iliac vessels that cross obliquely from the cranial to caudal and from the lateral to medial.

2.5.2 Laterally

Laterally, the relationship is the psoas muscle (and genitofemoral nerve), and also the infundibulopelvic ligament, with a parallel course.

2.5.3 Medially

Medially, the. Ureters are situated at 2 cm from the promontory.

2.5.4 Ventrally

Ventrally, on the right, the lower end of the mesentery, the ileocolic artery. The ileocecal angle and the appendix are lateral to its course.

On the left, the main relationship is the meso-sigmoid and the sigmoid arteries (upper, middle, lower) usually coming from the left colic artery.

2.6 Anatomical Relationships of the Pelvic Segment

The pelvic ureter follows the iliac segment from the pelvic brim to the bladder.

The ureter enters the pelvis after it crosses the iliac vessels. Generally, the right ureter crosses the external iliac artery, and the left ureter crosses the common iliac artery (Figs. 2.6 and 2.7). Then it passes dorsally and caudally on the pelvic wall under cover of the peritoneum. The ureter appears as a convex curve, especially at the level of the greater sciatic notch.

In the pelvis, the ureter lies below and forward of the internal iliac artery, crosses the medial side of the obturator nerve and vessels, and the umbilical artery (medial umbilical ligament).

The pelvic segment describes a concave curve in front, wherein we recognize two segments, one, parietal and the other, visceral.

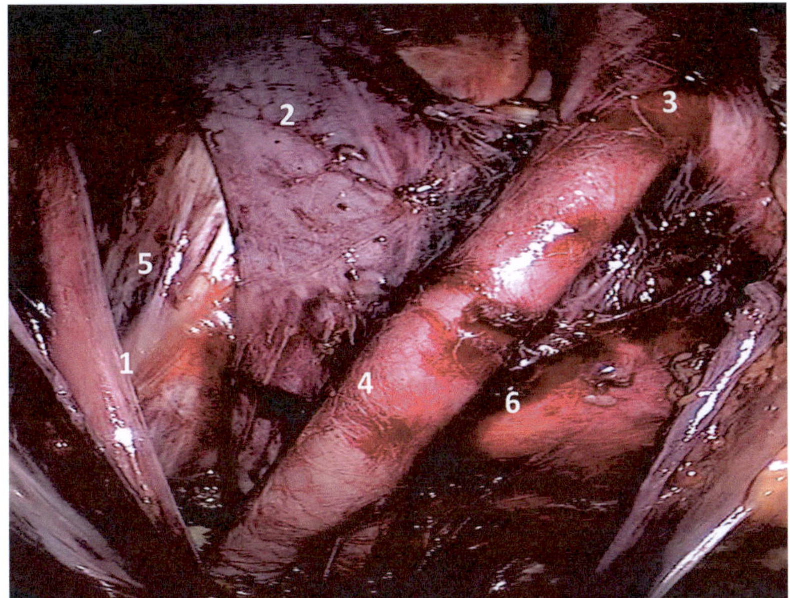

Fig. 2.4 Anatomical relationships of the iliac segment. Course of the ureter at the level of the promontory. Right side. Anatomic view. Dissection during laparoscopic paraaortic lymphadenectomy. (1) Ureter lateralized, (2) vena cava, (3) aortic bifurcation, (4) right common iliac artery, (5) psoas muscle, (6) promontory

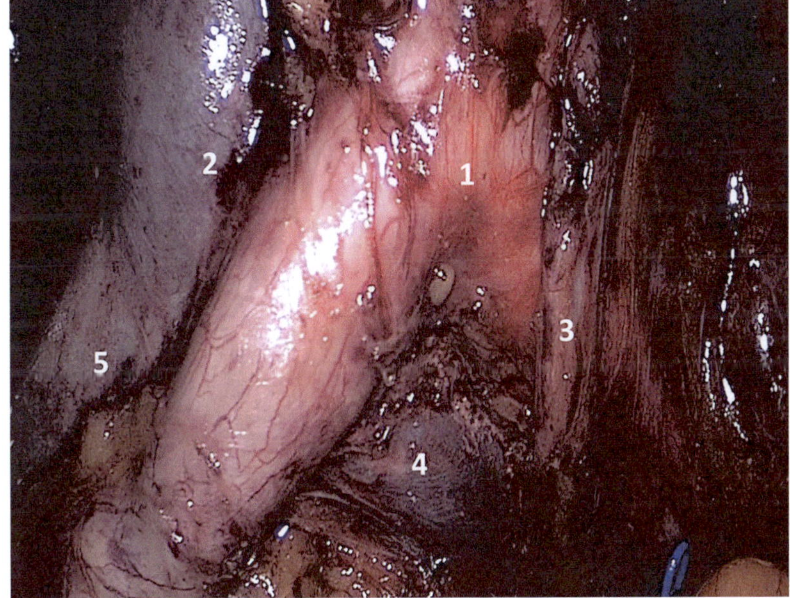

Fig. 2.5 Anatomical relationships of the iliac segment. Course of the ureter at the level of the promontory. Left side. Anatomic view. Dissection during laparoscopic paraaortic lymphadenectomy. (1) Aortic bifurcation, (2) vena cava, (3) left ureter, (4) left common iliac vein, (5) right common iliac vein

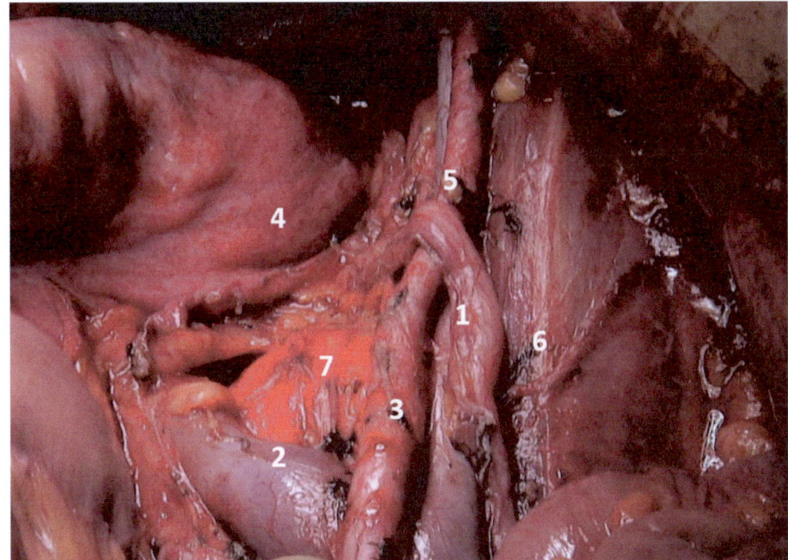

Fig. 2.6 Anatomical relationships of the iliac segment. Pelvic course of the ureter at the level of the iliac vessels. Right side. Superior view. Dissection during open paraaortic lymphadenectomy. (1) Ureter, (2) left common iliac vein, (3) right iliac common artery, (4) rectum, (5) external iliac vessels, (6) psoas muscle, (7) promontory

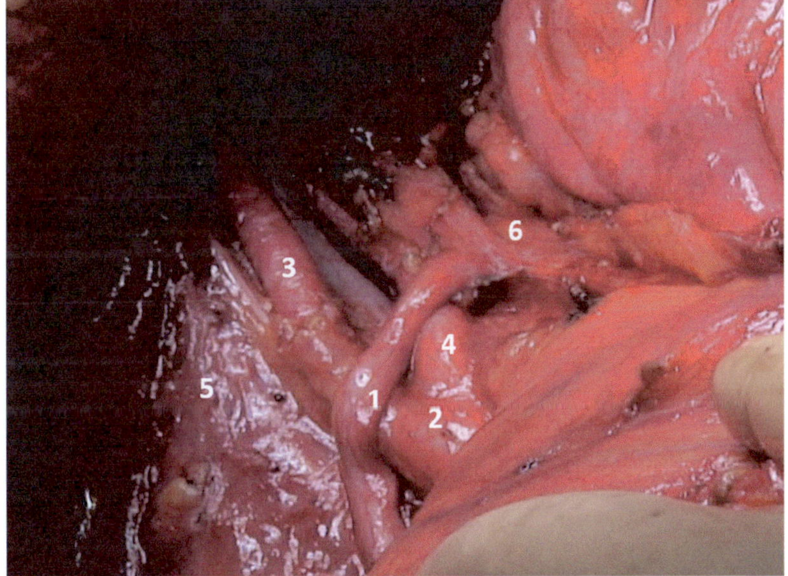

Fig. 2.7 Anatomical relationships of the iliac segment. Pelvic course of the ureter at the level of the iliac bifurcation. Left side. Superior view. Dissection during open paraaortic lymphadenectomy. (1) Ureter, (2) left common iliac bifurcation, (3) external iliac vessels, (4) internal iliac artery, (5) psoas, (6) rectum

2.6.1 Parietal Segment: Anterior Visualization of the Pelvic Segment (Fig. 2.8)

Figure 2.8 illustrates the anterior visualization of the pelvic segment of the ureter and the more posterior situation of the vaginal arteries.

Laterally, the relationships of the parietal segment are between the sciatic spine, the obturator vessels, and the superior vesical artery.

Medially, the peritoneum, the sheath of the internal iliac artery, and the hypogastric nerve.

Ventrally, the ovary, in forming the lower limit of the ovarian dimple. Then it descends laterally, medially to the ovarian vessels, and then down the anteromedial side of the uterine artery.

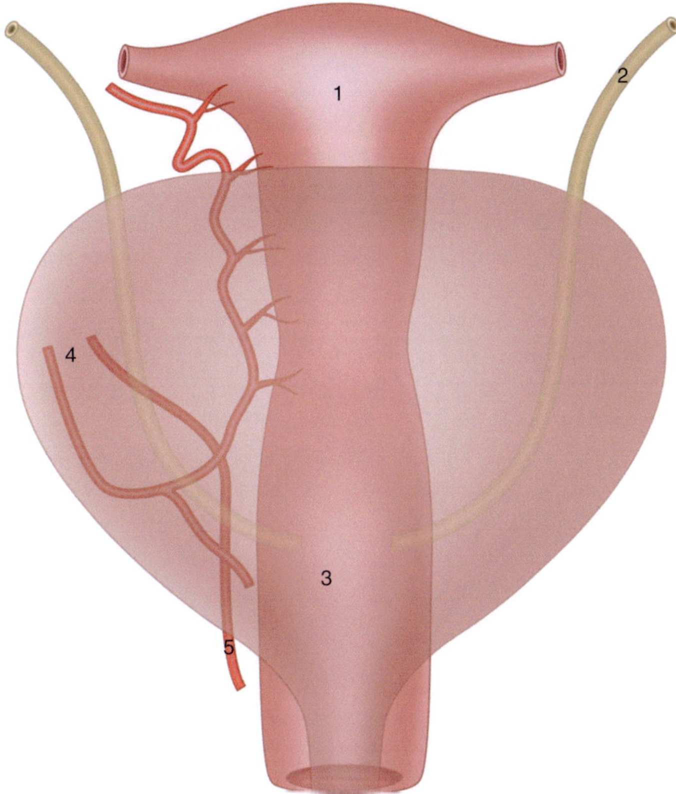

Fig. 2.8 Anterior visualization of the pelvic segment of the ureter. (1) Uterus, (2) ureter, (3) vagina, (4) uterine artery, (5) vaginal arteries (The bladder is represented in yellow shadow.)

2.6.2   Visceral Segment: Lateral Parametrium (Figs. 2.9 and 2.10)

The lower aspect of the ureter is surrounded by a dense plexus of veins communicating with the internal iliac vein. The terminal aspect of the ureter passes below the root of the broad ligament, through the Mackenrodt's ligament, and lies 2.0 cm lateral to the uterine cervix just above the lateral fornix of the vagina. Then it lies in front of the lateral margin of the vagina (Fig. 2.9).

In the Mackenrodt's ligament, the uterine artery and its small vein cross the ureter, passing forward and above. The ureteric branch of the uterine artery is located at the intersection, clearly visible when it exists. The main uterine vein lies behind the crossing. Then the ureter goes forward and inward with the cervicovaginal arterial and venous branches, the paracervix lymphatics, and the branches of the inferior hypogastric plexus and parasympathetic nerves. It is in contact with the Yabuki space, a small area between the uterus surface and the bladder surface (3). At this level, laterally, the vesicouterine ligament (and ureteric tunnel) contains the ureter (deep part of the bladder pillar). After a travel of about 1 cm, it enters the bladder on the posterior aspect of the trigone. In the end, the ureter is embedded within the bladder muscle for 1.9 cm (Fig. 2.10).

Fig. 2.9 Visceral segment of the ureter. Laparoscopic view on the left pelvic side wall. The visceral segment of the ureter engages under the broad ligament (Mackenrot's ligament). Main uterine veins are behind the crossing of the uterine artery and the ureter. Presumed ureteral course (red dashed lines). (1) Ovary, (2) uterine veins, (3) left ureter covered by the peritoneum, (4) uterosacral ligament, (5) Cul-de-sac of Douglas, (6) uterus

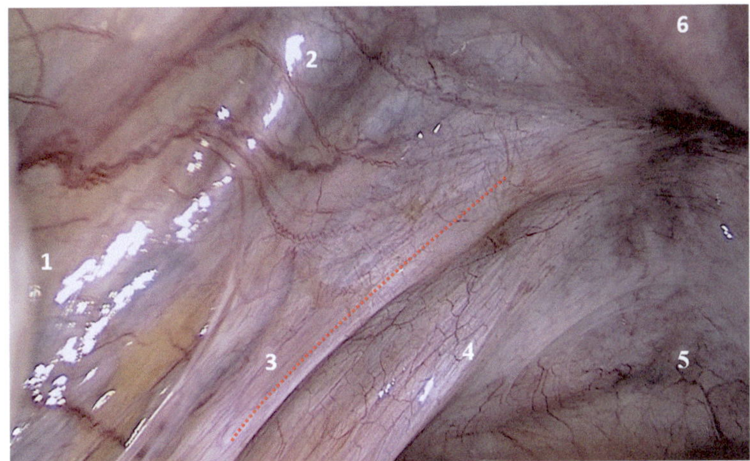

Fig. 2.10 Lateral parametrium. Left side. Dissection during laparoscopic radical hysterectomy. (1) Uterine artery, (2) ureter, (3) deep uterine vein, (4) ovary

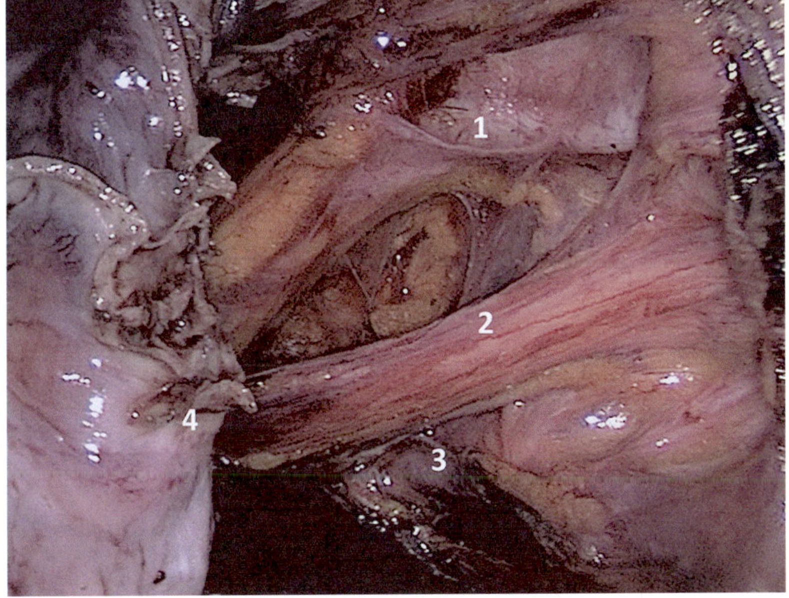

2.7   **Bladder Portion** (Fig. 2.11)

When the two ureters enter the bladder, they are 4 cm apart. They cross the wall obliquely downward and inward. The ureters end in the bladder two and a half centimeters apart. At the level of this connection, there is a mucous fold. When the bladder fills, urine will compress this fold and prevent backflow.

The ureter ends in a meatus, slightly narrowed and short.

2.8   **Anatomical Relationships of the Ureter and Pelvic Vessels** (Fig. 2.12)

Relationships between the ureter and pelvic vessels should be noted precisely.

The internal iliac artery divides itself into two trunks or divisions, anterior and posterior (respectively ventral and dorsal). The anterior trunk is visceral, giving obliterated umbilical artery, uterine artery, superior vesical artery, obturator artery, inferior vesical artery, middle rectal artery, internal pudendal artery, and inferior gluteal artery. The posterior trunk gives vessels that are far, lateral sacral artery, iliolumbar artery, and superior gluteal artery.

The main relationships of the ureter are the iliac arteries at the level of the promontory and the uterine artery at the level of the uterine isthmus.

Fig. 2.11 The bladder portion. Ureter entering into the bladder (vesicouterine ligament cut). Left side. Dissection during laparoscopic radical hysterectomy. (1) Ureter, (2) Yabuki space, (3) bladder, (4) vagina

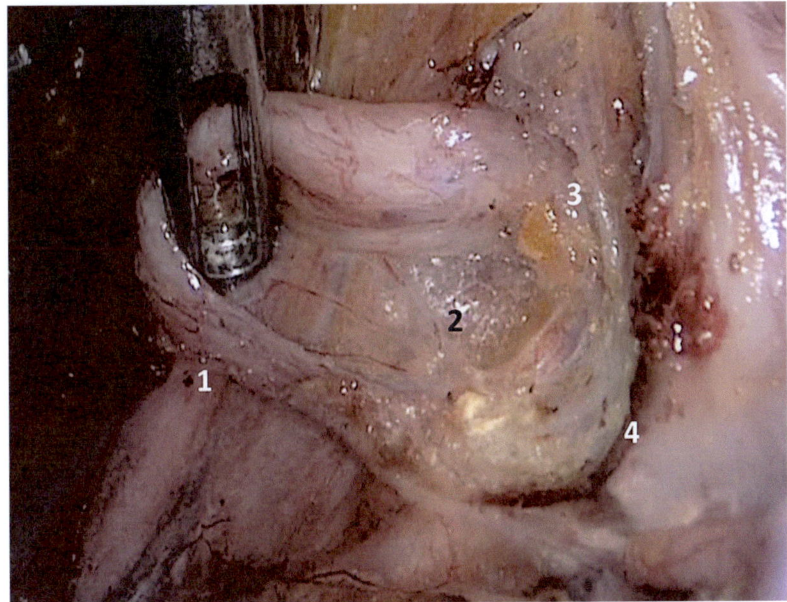

Fig. 2.12 Relationships between the ureter and pelvic vessels. We see the main vessels that we should localize according to the route of the ureter. (1) Ureter, (2) internal iliac artery, (3) external iliac artery, (4) obturator artery, (5) obliterated umbilical artery, (6) uterine artery, (7) inferior vesical artery, (8) middle rectal artery, (9) internal pudendal artery, (10) inferior gluteal artery

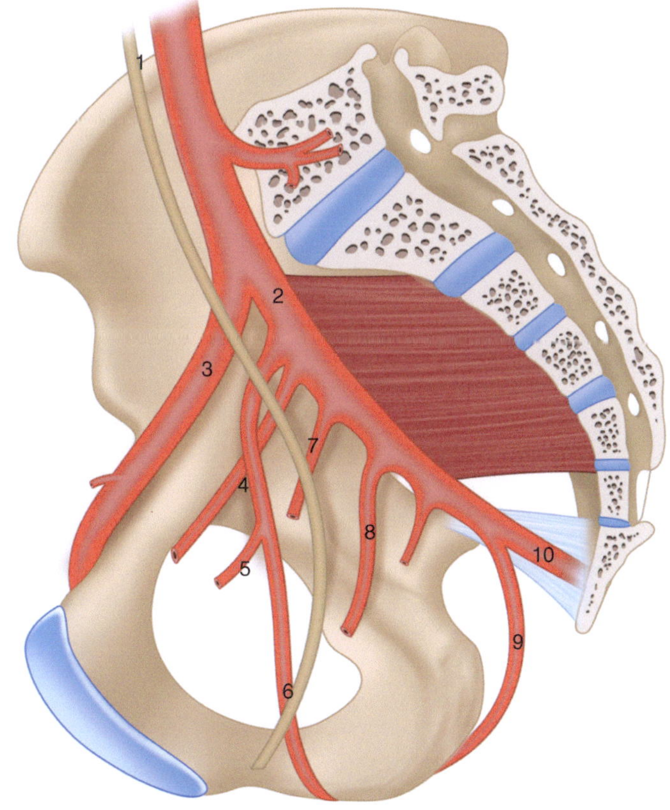

2.9 Cadaver Anatomy, Laparoscopic View of the Iliac Area (Fig. 2.13)

On the left side, the ureter crosses the common iliac artery and then takes its direction toward the pelvis.

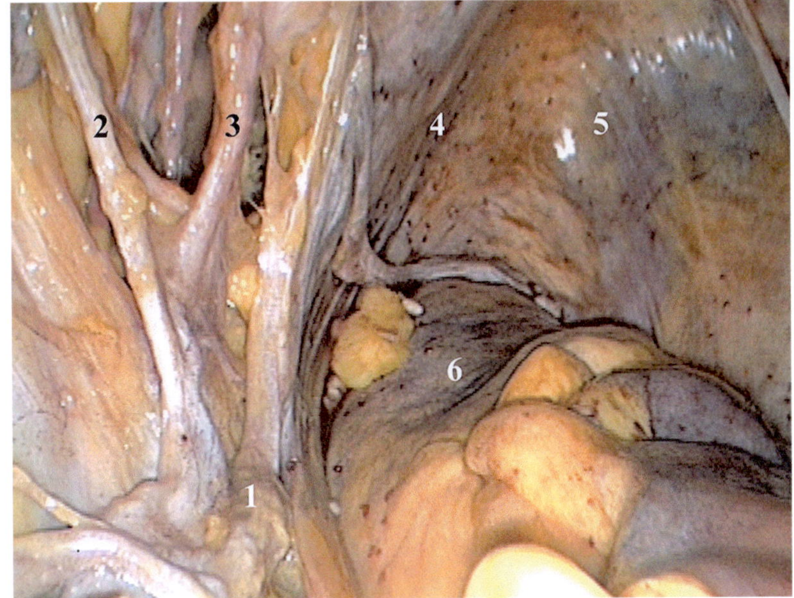

Fig. 2.13 Cadaver anatomy, ureter crossing the common iliac artery. Left side. (1) Ureter, (2) external iliac artery, (3) internal iliac artery, (4) uterosacral ligament, (5) Cul-de-sac of Douglas, (6) sigmoid bowel

References

1. Kamina P. Anatomie clinique, deuxième édition, Tome 4. Maloine; 2008. p. 33–43.

2. Puntambekar S, Manchanda R. Surgical pelvic anatomy in gynecologic oncology. Int J Gynecol Obstet. 2018;143(52):86–92.

Generalities on the Ureter

3

© The Author(s), under exclusive license to Springer Nature Switzerland AG 2022
J.-B. Dubuisson et al., *Ureteral Complications of Gynecological Surgery*,
https://doi.org/10.1007/978-3-031-15598-7_3

Chapter 3 describes the main characteristics of the ureter, and its usefulness for the pelvic surgeon: segmental vascularization, innervation, congenital anomalies, and histology.

3.1 Segmental Vascularization (Fig. 3.1)

The vascularization is segmental, provided by the ureteric arteries.

In its upper part, it receives its vascularization from the renal arteries.

In its middle part, from the aorta, the ovarian artery, and the common iliac artery.

At its lower part, from branches of the internal iliac artery, the vesical artery, the middle rectal artery, and the uterine artery.

Each ureteric artery divides into two branches as soon as it reaches the ureter to form an anastomotic network at the level of the adventitia. Then these branches penetrate the muscle to the mucosa.

3.2 Nerves

Nerves from T12 to L2 provide sympathetic afferent innervation creating a ureteral plexus. They originate from the renal, ovarian, and hypogastric plexuses. Pain refers to T12-L2 dermatomes. Efferent fibers originate from the sympathetic and parasympathetic ganglia. All of these are in the adventitia and must be preserved during any dissection.

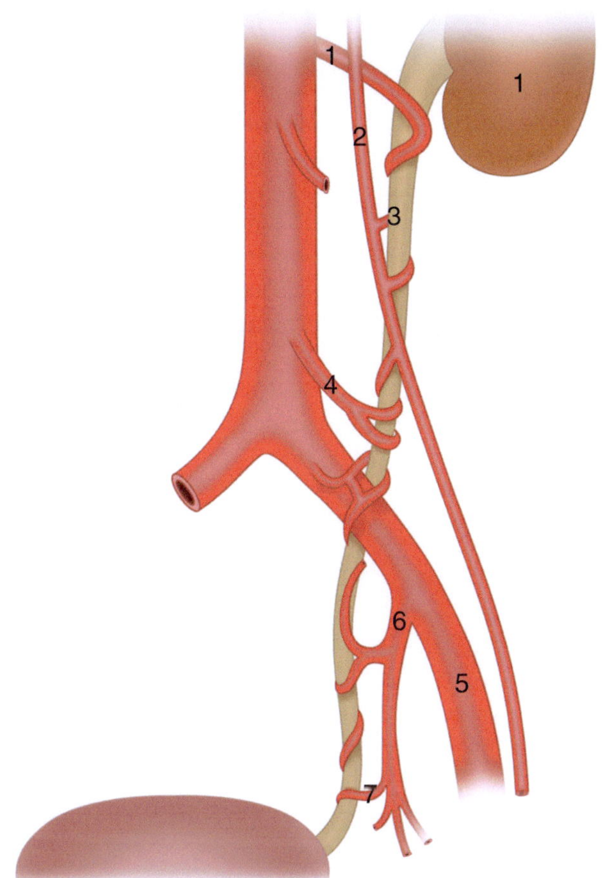

Fig. 3.1 Segmental vascularization of the ureter. The vascularization is segmental, provided by several ureteric arteries. For the gynecologist, the lower part is the most interesting. For this part, vessels are branches of internal iliac, vesical, uterine, and middle rectal arteries, organized at the level of the adventitia as a "mesoureter." (1) Kidney and renal vessels, (2) ovarian artery, (3) ureter, (4) inferior mesenteric artery, (5) external iliac artery, (6) internal iliac artery, (7) uterine artery

3.3   Congenital Anomalies
(Figs. 3.2, 3.3, 3.4, 3.5, 3.6 and 3.7)

There is a great variety of congenital anomalies.

Supernumerary ureters and abnormal terminations may be observed.

Unilateral duplication or duplicity involves two ureters that end in two ostia in the bladder.

When we see two ureters on one side, a supernumerary kidney, or a blind-ending of one of the ureters can be observed.

The unilateral ureteral bifidity corresponds to two ureters that unite with a single vesical ostium.

The horseshoe may be seen.

The agenesis is very rare.

The congenital hypoplasia of the ureter is rare and associated with hypoplasia of the kidney.

The megalo-ureter and angulation and rotation (corkscrew ureter) may be observed.

The diverticulum may occur at any part of the ureter but especially at the ureteropelvic junction, near the crossing with the iliac artery, and at the ureterovesical junction.

The retrocaval ureter is limited to the right side.

Fig. 3.2 Urinary tract malformation: right duplex kidney. Incomplete fusion of the upper and lower pole of the kidney which creates two separate drainage systems from the kidney. Coronal reconstruction from CT in delayed phase demonstrating the low position of the right kidney with two urinary ureters (red arrow) and collecting systems

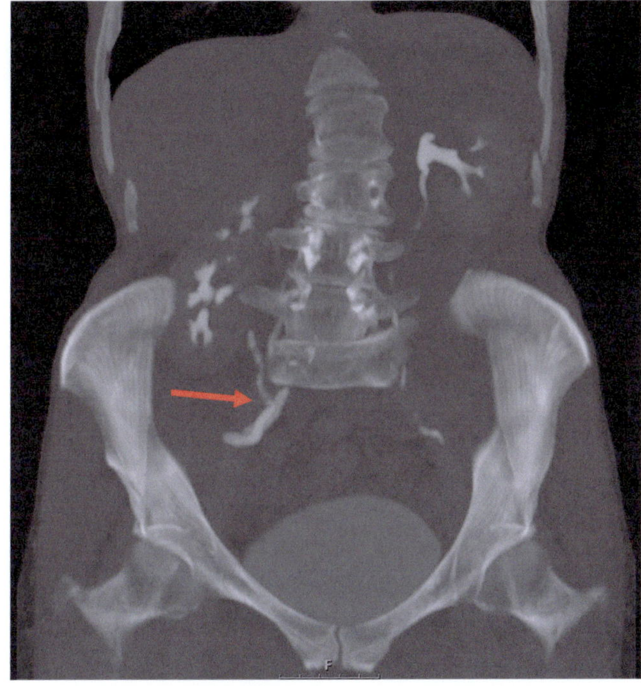

Fig. 3.3 Right duplex kidney with duplicated collecting system. Red arrow: visualization of two ureteral sites of implantation at the level of the vesicoureteral junction

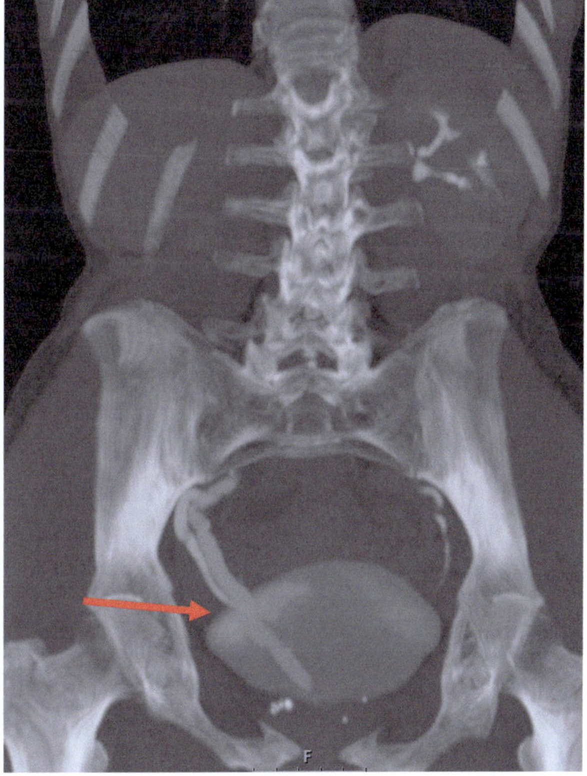

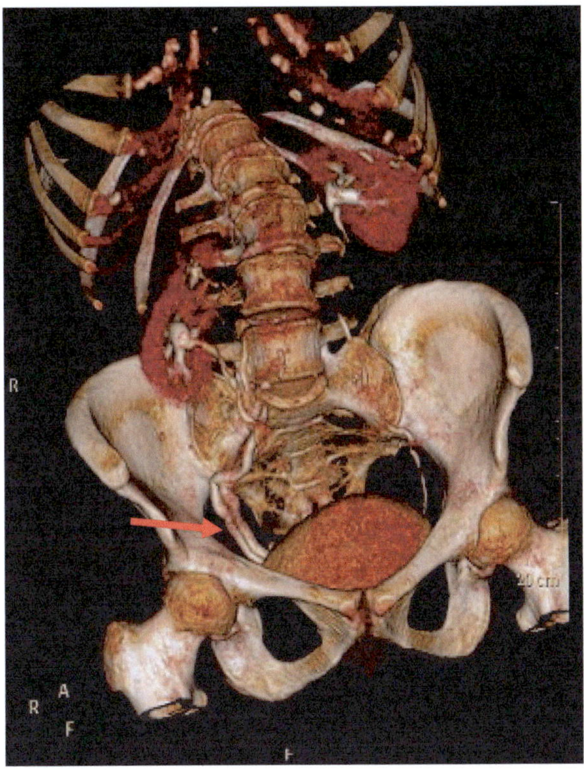

Fig. 3.4 Right duplex kidney. CT-scan with 3D reconstruction. Red arrow: duplicated collecting system

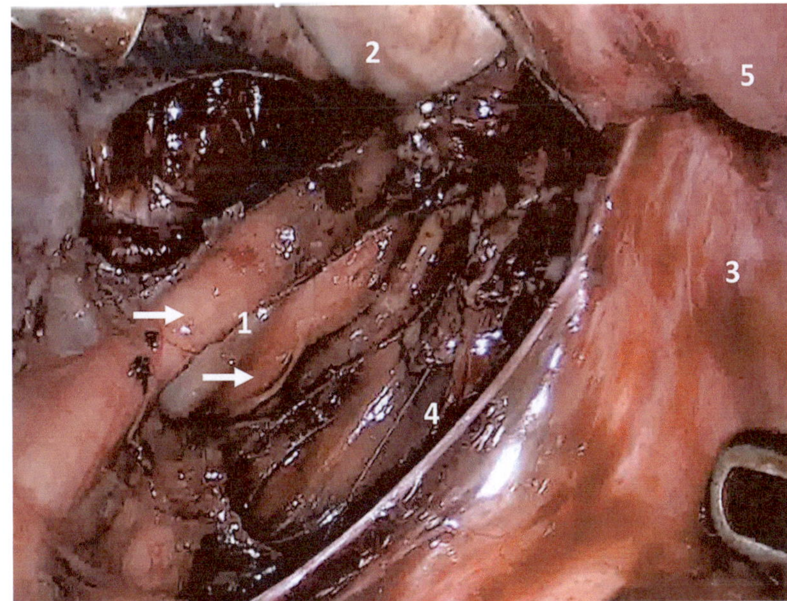

Fig. 3.5 Congenital anomalies. Ureteral duplication. Left side. Laparoscopic dissection for deep infiltrating endometriosis. (1) Ureters (white arrows), (2) ovary, (3) left uterosacral ligament with endometriotic lesions, (4) medial pararectal space (Okabayashi space), (5) uterus

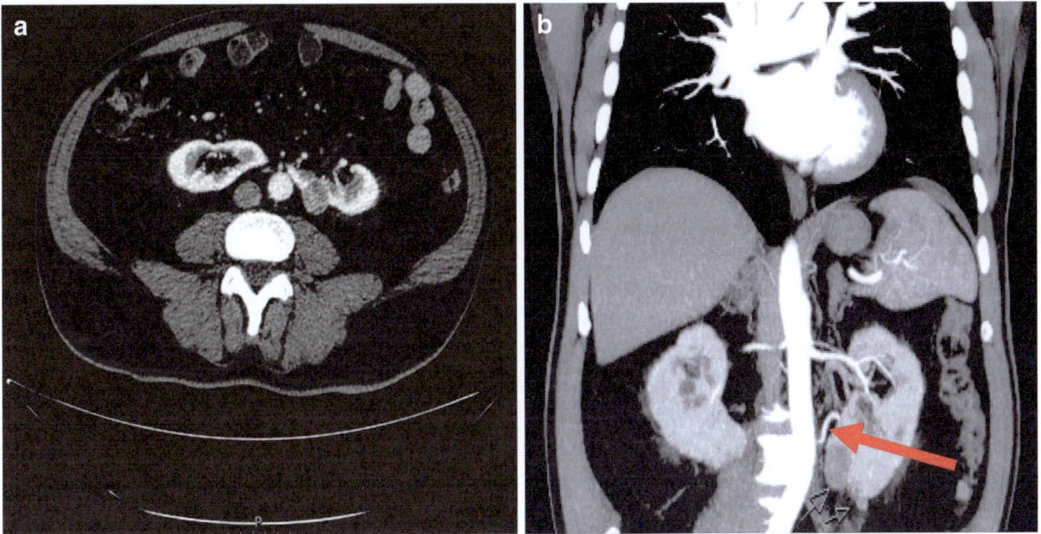

Fig. 3.6 Horseshoe kidney. Axial (**a**) and coronal view (**b**) with vascular variation: two polar renal arteries (red arrow)

Fig. 3.7 Right kidney
agenesia. CT-scan:
coronal reconstruction

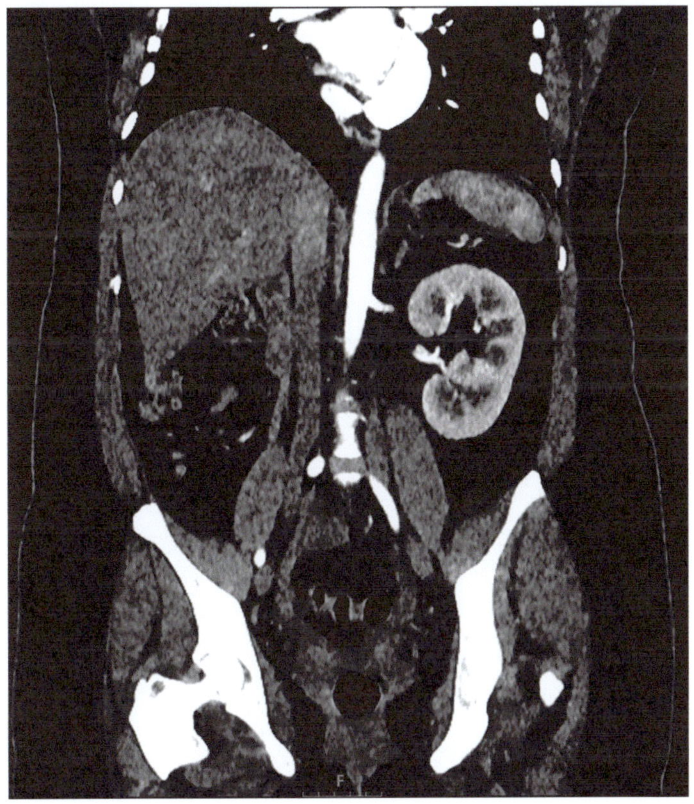

3.4 Histology (Fig. 3.8)

The ureter is intimately linked to the peritoneum, which comprises the outside to the inside of the three main structures.

3.4.1 Adventitia

This loose fibroelastic connective tissue with vessels and nerves constitutes the ureteric sheath (or Waldeyer's).

3.4.2 Muscular Layer

The detrusor, smooth muscle fibers, is made up of two rather plexiform layers (internal longitudinal and external circular) that allow the progression of urine through their coordinated crawling movement. A thicker layer of longitudinal fibers was observed in the lower part.

3.4.3 Mucosa

The mucosa or urothelium (polymorphic pseudostratified epithelium with 4–6 layers thick) forms folds and the underlying chorion or lamina propria contains nerves and vessels. Its lower end has the Waldeyer's sheath with longitudinal fibers forming an anti-regurgitation valve.

3.4.4 Activity of the Ureter

Urine transport is by bolus due to peristaltic waves. Urine is ejected into the bladder at a rate varying from 1 to 6 per minute.

Fig. 3.8 Histology of the ureter. It includes from outside to inside: The conjunctivo-elastic tunica (adventitia) with vessels, nerves; the muscular or detrusor: with two layers (internal longitudinal and external circular); the mucosa or urothelium (polymorphic pseudostratified epithelium) with folds and the underlying chorion or lamina propria containing nerves and vessels. (1) Adventitial tissue, (2) circular muscle, (3) longitudinal muscle, (4) epithelium, (5) lamina propria, (6) arteries

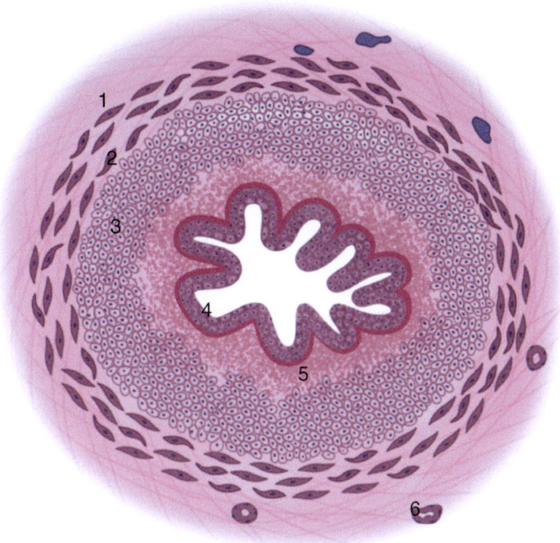

Different Anatomical Aspects of the Ureter in Laparoscopy

4

J.-B. Dubuisson et al., *Ureteral Complications of Gynecological Surgery*,
https://doi.org/10.1007/978-3-031-15598-7_4

Chapter 4 concerns full and comprehensive description of the different aspects of the ureter in laparoscopy: relationships between ureter and promontory, iliac arteries, infundibulopelvic ligament, ovarian fossa, uterosacral ligament, hypogastric nerve, uterine vessels, entry in the Mackenrodt's ligament, and entry in the bladder [1, 2].

4.1 Relationship Between Ureter and Promontory (Fig. 4.1)

There is a risk of injury of the ureter at the level of the promontory. On both sides, the risk exists during difficult surgeries of the adnexa. We should mention the ovarian tumors, and the severe adhesions modifying the usual anatomy, especially in cases of deep infiltrating endometriosis.

On the left side, the risk exists in cases of colorectal pathologies and corresponding surgeries. On the right side, during sacrocolpopexy, it is necessary to well identify the ureter before fixing the mesh to the anterior longitudinal ligament covering the promontory.

4.2 Ureter and Iliac Arteries in Laparoscopy (Figs. 4.2 and 4.3)

The bifurcation of the internal iliac artery from a common iliac artery is at the level of the sacral promontory. The internal iliac artery is visible when the peritoneum is thin and transparent. To know its background, the peritoneum must be incised with dissections of the different spaces. Internal iliac arteries go downward and medially and divide after 2–3 cm.

One of the easiest places to find the ureter is to focus on the common iliac artery and its bifurcation. It is sometimes less easy to find it on the left side because of the volume of the sigmoid colon or in case of obesity (Fig. 4.2).

During peristaltic movements, the ureter is well visible through the peritoneum, taking a pearly white color (Fig. 4.3).

Fig. 4.1 Relationship between ureter and promontory. Right side. (1) Promontory, (2) ureter, (3) external iliac artery, (4) presacral vessels, (5) bowel

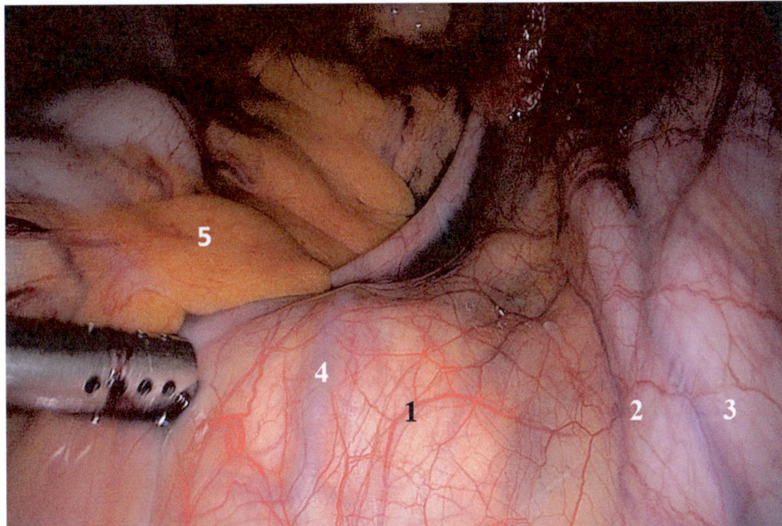

Fig. 4.2 Ureter and iliac arteries. Right side. (1) Psoas muscle, (2) genitofemoral nerve, (3) ureter, (4) bowel, (5) common iliac artery, (6) infundibulopelvic ligament, (7) uterosacral ligament, (8) fallopian tube

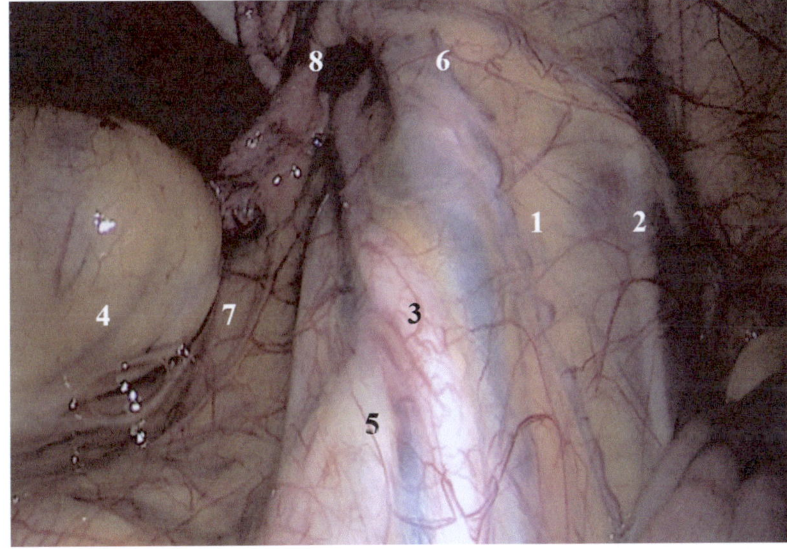

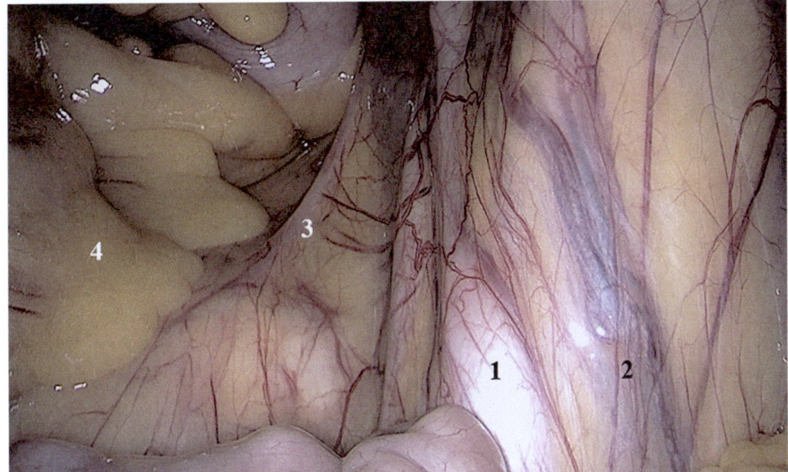

Fig. 4.3 Ureter and iliac arteries. Peristalsis of the ureter. Right side. (1) Crawl of the ureter. Ureter crossing iliac vessels, (2) infundibulopelvic ligament, (3) uterosacral ligament, (4) bowel

4.3   Ureter and Infundibulopelvic Ligament, in Laparoscopy
(Figs. 4.4, 4.5, 4.6, 4.7 and 4.8)

After the crossing of the iliac vessels, the ureter is always below the infundibulopelvic ligament containing ovarian vessels, usually at 3–4 cm. The ureter may be covered by fat tissue, especially in obese women (Fig. 4.4).

The peritoneal fold allows us to spot it (Fig. 4.5).

Usually, the distance between the two organs is evident, especially after the tension of the infundibulopelvic ligament (Fig. 4.6).

Sometimes, the distance between the infundibulopelvic ligament and the ureter is shorter (Fig. 4.7).

The lateral approach for oncologic surgery consists of a longitudinal peritoneal incision lateral to the infundibulopelvic ligament which gives immediate access to the external iliac artery.

The medial approach for endometriosis surgery consists of a peritoneal incision medial to the infundibulopelvic ligament. This incision gives access to the ureter just under the peritoneum after a short dissection of the internal iliac artery.

The panoramic view when during vNOTES (vaginal Natural Orifice Transluminal Endoscopic Surgery) procedures should be mentioned. The view of the ureter and the infundibulopelvic ligament is as the classical vision through the vaginal access: the view is reversed. The infundibulopelvic ligament and the ovarian pedicle are "above" the ureter. The ureter runs ventrally (Fig. 4.8).

Fig. 4.4 Ureter and infundibulopelvic ligament. Right side. The ureter is always below the ovarian vessels, usually at a distance of 3–4 cm. (1) Ureter, (2) infundibulopelvic ligament, (3) bowel, (4) right ovary

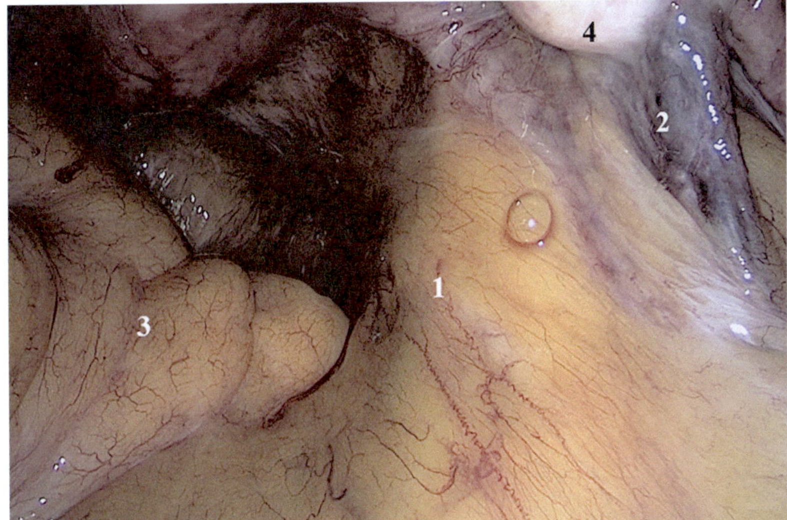

Fig. 4.5 Ureter and infundibulopelvic ligaments. Right side. The peritoneal fold of the ureter is well seen. (1) Ovary, (2) psoas muscle, (3) ovarian pedicle, (4) ureter, (5) fallopian tube, (6) bowel

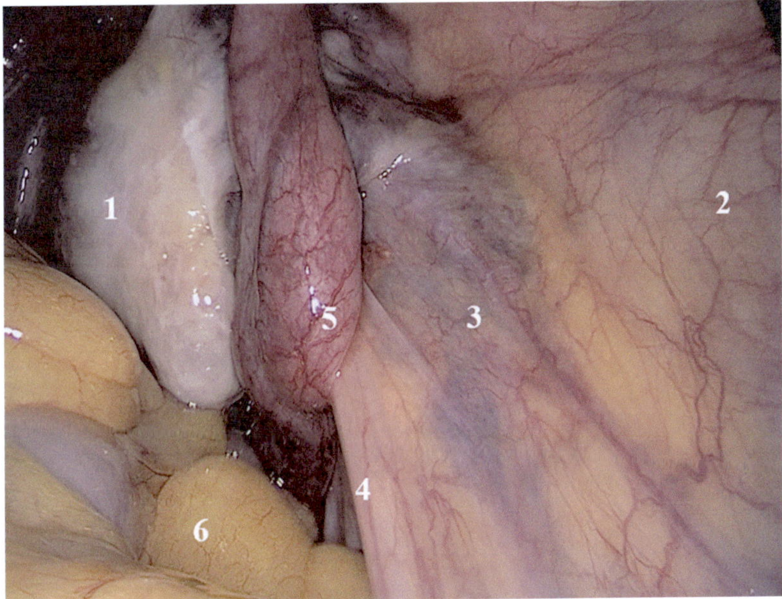

Fig. 4.6 Ureter and infundibulopelvic ligament. Distance between the two organs. Pulling up the adnexa with a forceps, the ureter is away from the ureter. Second-look 3 months after total hysterectomy. Right side. (1) Cul-de-sac of Douglas, (2) uterosacral ligament, (3) ureter, (4) infundibulopelvic ligament, (5) internal iliac artery

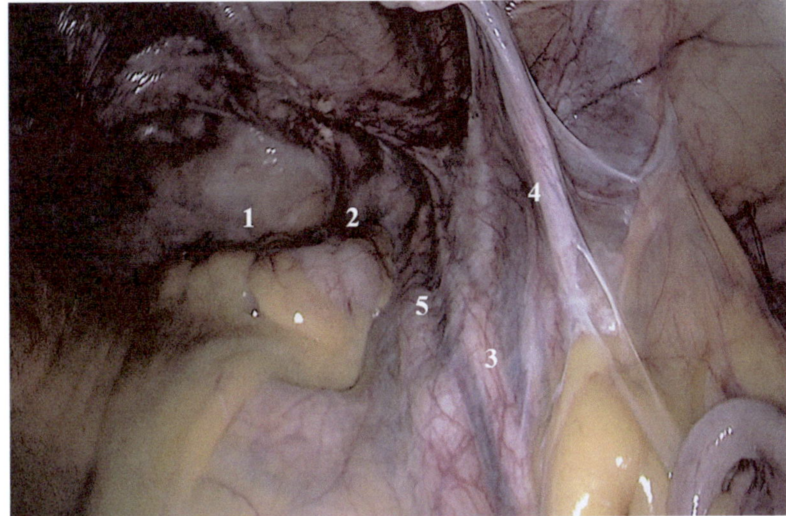

Fig. 4.7 Ureter and infundibulopelvic ligament. Short distance between ureter and ovarian pedicle in this case. Right side. (1) Ovary, (2) psoas muscle, (3) infundibulopelvic ligament, (4) ureter, (5) common iliac artery, (6) uterosacral ligament, (7) Douglas cul-de-sac, (8) rectum

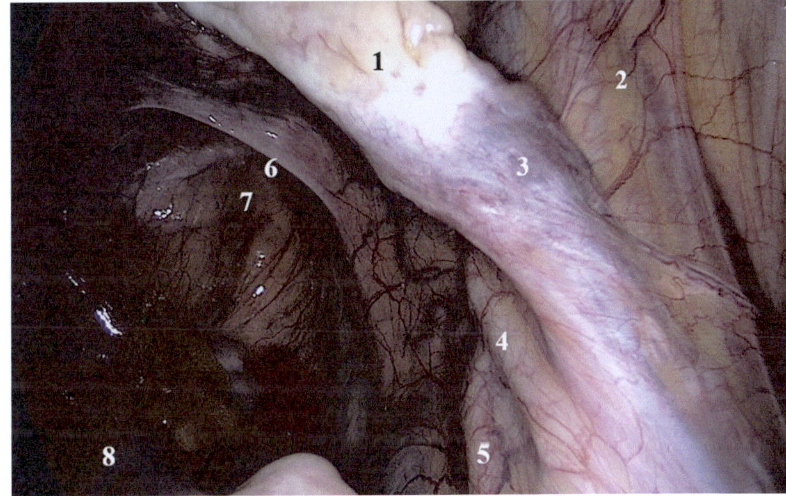

Fig. 4.8 vNOTES view
of the ureter and the
uterosacral ligament.
Right side. (1) Ureter,
(2) infundibulopelvic
ligament, (3) bowel

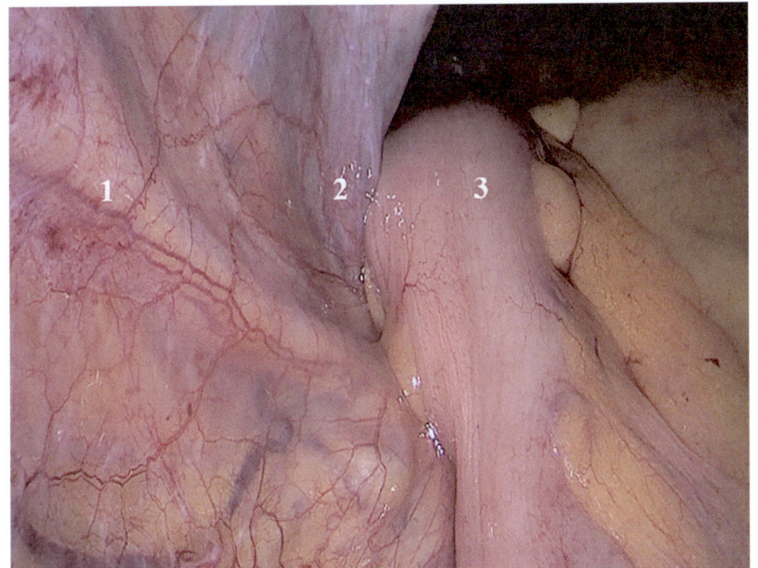

4.4 Ureter and Ovarian Fossa, in Laparoscopy (Figs. 4.9, 4.10, 4.11, and 4.12)

The ovarian fossa is a depression on the lateral wall where the ovary lays on. Its boundaries are superiorly external iliac artery, obliterated umbilical artery, and inferiorly to the ureter. The main peritoneal folds around the ovary and its fossa are well defined. This proximity explains well that adhesions due to severe endometriosis or ovarian malignancy may affect the ureter, at the level of the fossa (Fig. 4.9).

A shallow ovarian fossa may be observed. The morphology of the ovarian fossa is very variable from side to side and from woman to woman. In Fig. 4.10, there is a large distance between the three organs (Fig. 4.10).

In patients with a large ovarian cyst, free of adhesions, the ovary leaves its fossa and lays on the cul-de-sac of Douglas or above the uterus (Fig. 4.11).

In patients with fixed endometrioma, the ureter is sometimes very close, hidden by adhesions (Fig. 4.12).

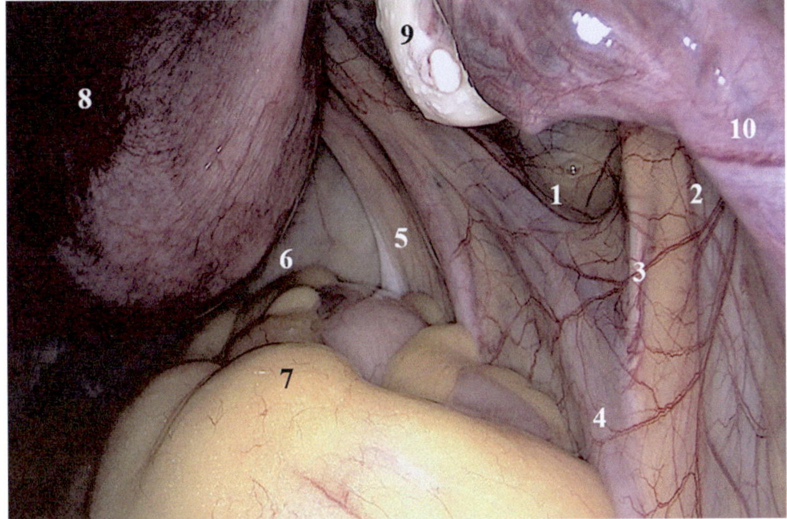

Fig. 4.9 Ureter and ovarian fossa. Right side. Laparoscopic view. (1) Ovarian fossa, (2) external iliac vein, (3) umbilical artery, 4) ureter, (5) uterosacral ligament, 6) cul-de-sac of Douglas, (7) bowel, (8) uterus, 9) ovary, (10) infundibulopelvic ligament

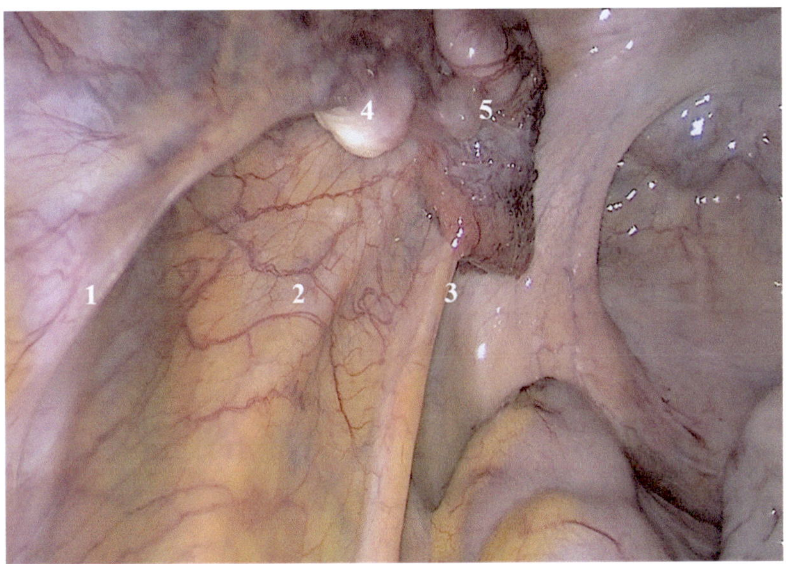

Fig. 4.10 Ureter and ovarian fossa. Left side. A shallow ovarian fossa. (1) Infundibulopelvic ligament, (2) ureter, (3) uterosacral ligament, (4) ovary, (5) tube

Fig. 4.11 Ureter and ovarian fossa. Right side. In patients with large ovarian cyst, free of adhesions, the ovary leaves its fossa to stay on the cul-de-sac of Douglas or above the uterus. (1) Ureter, (2) uterosacral ligament, (3) ovarian fossa, (4) tube, (5) infundibulopelvic ligament, (6) right ovarian cyst

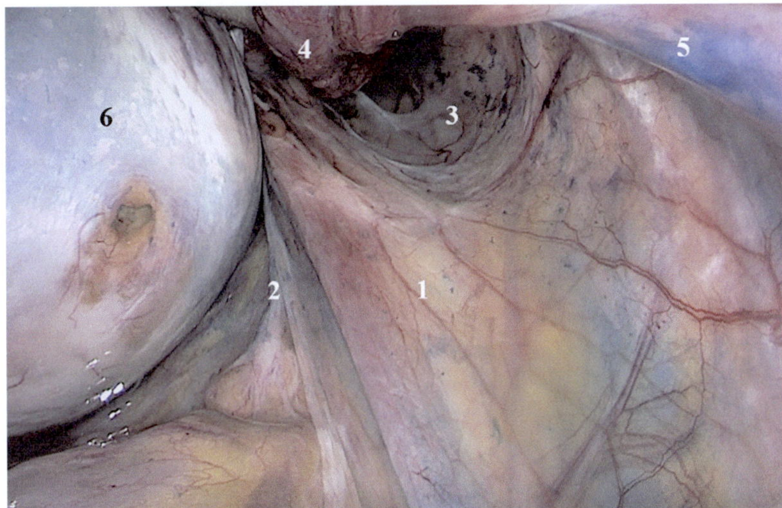

Fig. 4.12 Ureter and ovarian fossa. Right side. (1) Ureter, (2) ovarian fossa, (3) infundibulopelvic ligament, (4) uterosacral ligament, (5) fixed ovary in the fossa, (6) cul-de-sac of Douglas

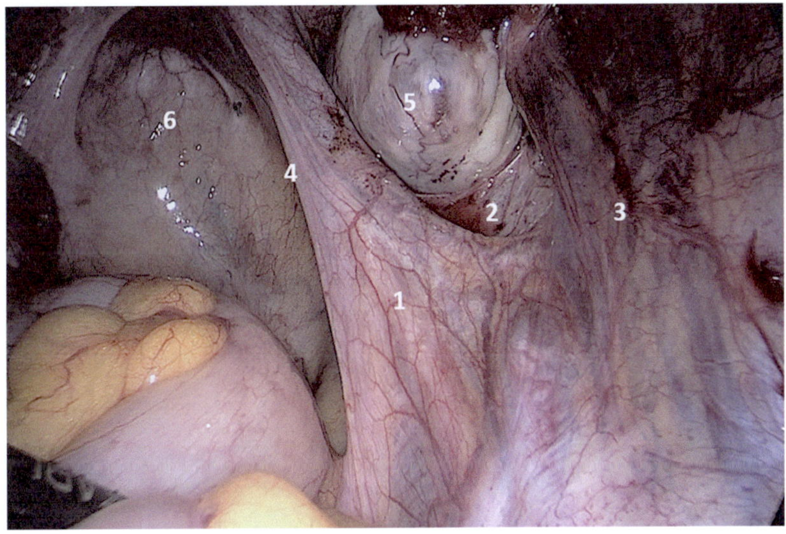

4.5   Ureter and Uterosacral Ligaments (Figs. 4.13, 4.14 and 4.15)

The uterosacral ligaments are located between the presacral fascia dorsally and the torus of the uterus ventrally. Usually, they are well identified when the uterus is pushed ventrally during laparoscopy. At its dorsal part, and at the level of the infundibulopelvic ligament, the uterosacral ligament is quite far from the ureter (Fig. 4.13).

At its ventral part, the uterosacral ligament gets closer to the ureter (Fig. 4.14).

How to get away from the ureter at the level of the ovarian fossa? Gripping the uterosacral ligament and pushing it medially moves the ureter away. It gives more safety to removing the posterior endometriotic nodule of the uterosacral ligaments and dissecting the ovary from the ovarian fossa (Fig. 4.15).

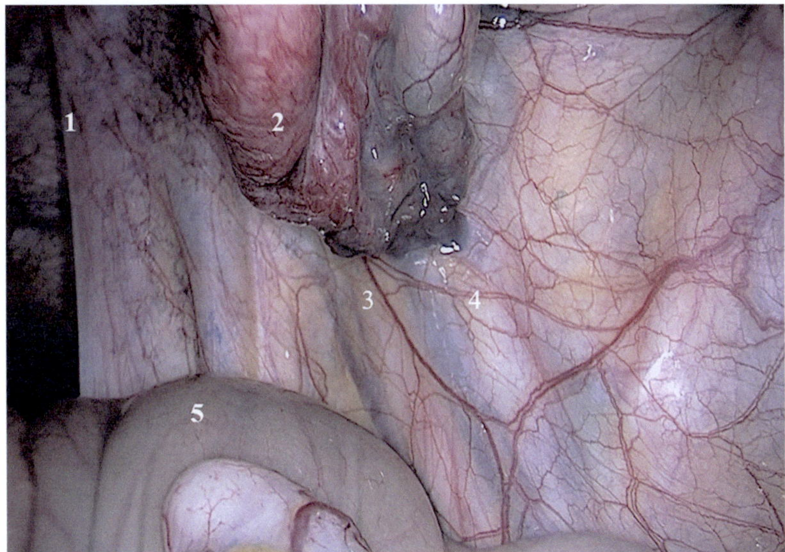

Fig. 4.13 Ureter and uterosacral ligament. The uterosacral ligaments are situated between the presacral fascia and the torus uterinum. The dorsal part of the ligament is quite far from the ureter. (1) Uterosacral ligament, (2) tube, (3) ureter, (4) uterine vessels, (5) small intestine

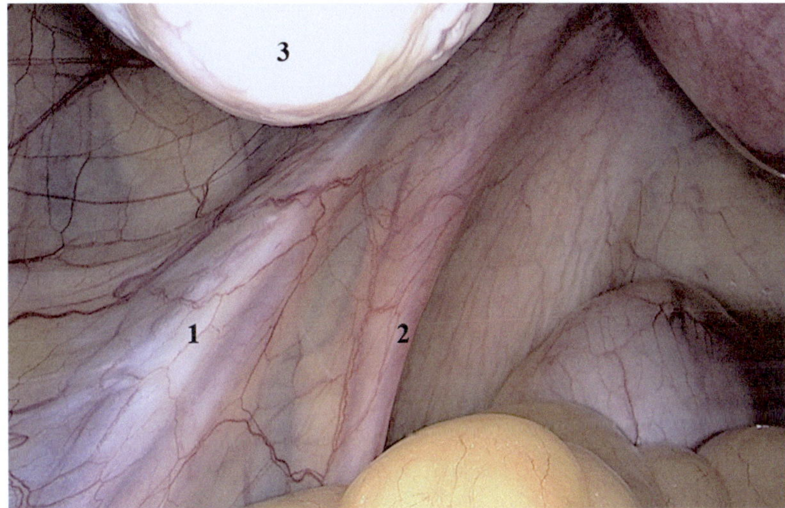

Fig. 4.14 Ureter and uterosacral ligaments: the approximation close to the torus uterinum. Left side. (1) Ureter, (2) uterosacral ligament, (3) ovary

Fig. 4.15 Ureter and uterosacral ligament, during operative strategy. Necessity to get away from the ureter. In this case, proximity of uterosacral ligament and ureter. Left side. (1) Ureter, (2) uterine vessels, (3) uterosacral ligament, (4) cul-de-sac of Douglas

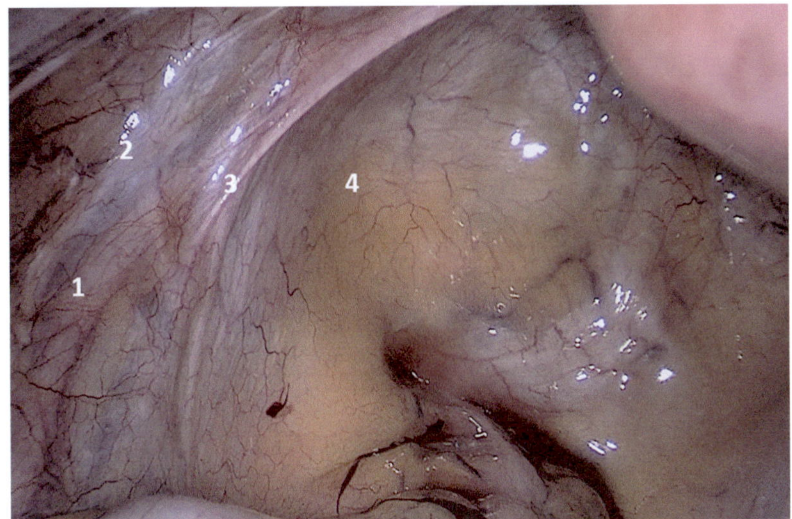

4.6 Ureter and Hypogastric Nerve (Figs. 4.16 and 4.17)

The hypogastric nerve is located in the pararectal space, lateral to the rectum, and the medial part of the pararectal space (Okabayashi space). It connects the superior hypogastric plexus to the inferior hypogastric plexus (Fig. 4.16).

It is between the uterosacral ligament and the ureter.

The nerve lies deep at the base of the uterosacral ligament. Then, it is often seen just under the peritoneum, always lateral to the uterosacral ligament. During surgery, remaining the medial to the uterosacral ligament will avoid damage to the nerve. It is located at 2 cm under the ureter. Finally, the hypogastric nerve crosses the uterosacral ligament at 3 cm from the torus uterinum.

Usually, there is a distance between the uterosacral ligament, hypogastric nerve, and ureter (Fig. 4.17).

Fig. 4.16 Ureter and hypogastric nerve. Description. Right side. (1) Fallopian tube, (2) ovary, (3) ovarian fossa, (4) cul-de-sac of Douglas, (5) uterosacral ligament, (6) hypogastric nerve, (7) ureter, (8) bowel, (9) obliterated umbilical artery

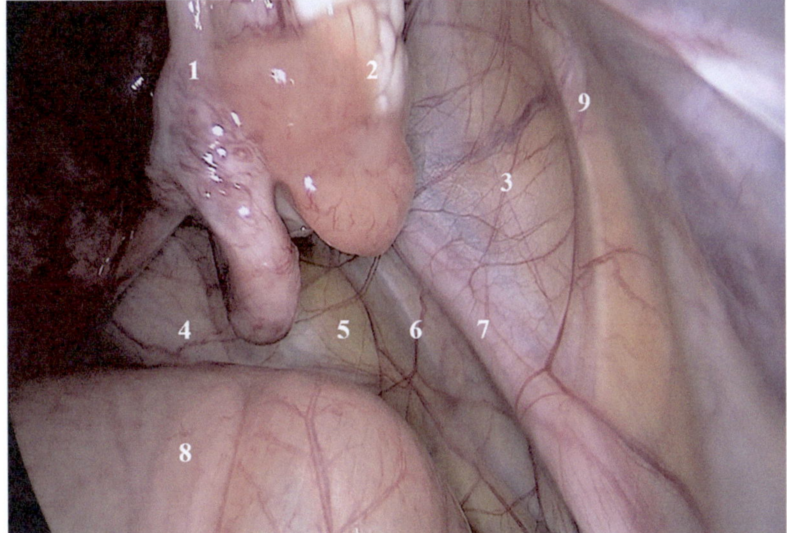

Fig. 4.17 Ureter and hypogastric nerve. The distance. Right side. (1) Tube, (2) ovary, (3) ovarian fossa, (4) cul-de-sac of Douglas, (5) uterosacral ligament, (6) hypogastric nerve, (7) ureter, (8) infundibulopelvic ligament, (9) common iliac vessels, (10) bowel

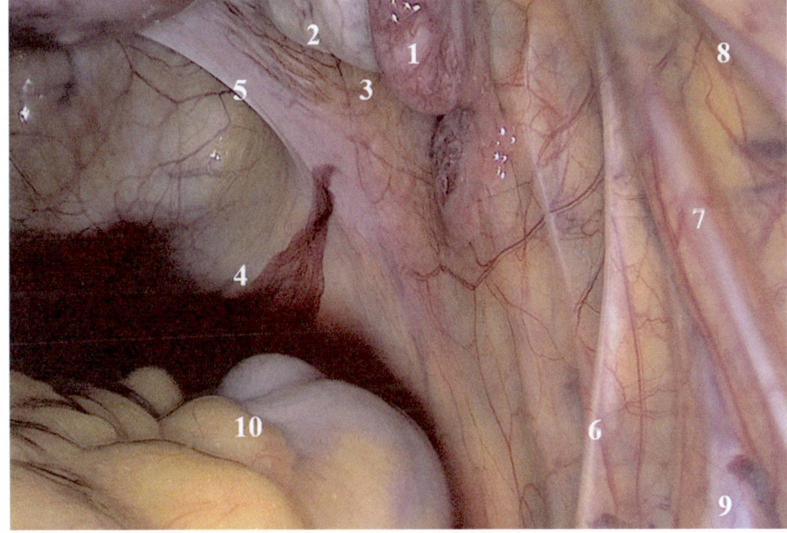

## 4.7	Ureter and Uterine Vessels in Laparoscopy (Figs. 4.18 and 4.19)

It is fundamental to distinguish clearly the internal iliac artery and uterine artery. Which may not be evident in the case of intraoperative bleeding. The internal iliac artery divides into two trunks or divisions (anterior and posterior). The division is situated 2–3 cm distal to the division of the common iliac artery. The anterior trunk continues usually through the medial umbilical ligament and gives many branches on the medial and lateral sides of the pelvis. The first main branch is usually the uterine artery which arises 5–6 cm distal to the origin of the posterior division. Several variations of the anterior trunk have been described. The uterine artery may be a separate branch of the internal iliac artery. It may be a common trunk with the medial umbilical ligament, or with the inferior gluteal artery. Trifurcation with superior and inferior arteries has been described.

Concerning the internal iliac artery, the segment of the anterior trunk between the origin of the posterior trunk and the branch of the uterine artery is usually free of other branches and may be easily located at laparoscopy. Just 1–2 cm proximal to the origin of the uterine artery the internal iliac artery may be easily dissected from the internal iliac vein without risk of bleeding, and it is the best place for ligation of the internal iliac artery in case of uterine or vaginal hemorrhage during delivery. The internal iliac artery forms the lateral boundary of paravesical and pararectal space which are connected from under the peritoneum. They are divided by the uterine artery.

The ureter has no relation with the paravesical space. It has relationships with the pararectal space.

The pararectal space is explored after surgical dissection. The incision of the peritoneum at the level of the sacral promontory is safe for the ureter and the pararectal space may be reached. It is divided by the ureter in two spaces, lateral and medial.

The lateral pararectal space or Latzko space is a pyramid whose base is the levator ani muscle, and the peak is at the level at which the ureter crosses the common iliac artery. The uterine artery crosses the space transversely with below parasympathetic nerves. It can be ligated in the pararectal space. It lies above the ureter. But the uterine vein is below the ureter and may bleed in case of a deep dissection.

The medial pararectal space or Okabayashi space is bordered laterally by the ureter and medially by the uterosacral ligament. The main structures seen inside are the hypogastric nerve which courses longitudinally and the uterine vein which crosses transversely toward the Latzko space.

In summary, lateral to the rectum, from medial to lateral, the structures are Okabayashi space, ureter, Latzko space, internal iliac artery, and above the transversely uterine artery.

We must mention the Yabuki space which is the triangular space seen between the uterus surface, the bladder, and the anterior vesicouterine ligament (or ureteric tunnel). It contains ureter and splanchnic nerves.

In some patients, there is dangerous proximity between the umbilical ligament and the uterine artery forming sometimes a trunk, and the internal iliac artery. We follow the right internal iliac artery with its descent from top to bottom, medial to the ureter. The crossing of the ureter with the uterine artery is still far away (Fig. 4.18).

Concerning cohabitation with other pelvic organs, Fig. 4.19 illustrates the classical view of the laparoscopic anatomy with the usual situation of the bowel in the pelvic cavity in case of low CO_2 pressure and limited Trendelenburg position (Fig. 4.19).

Fig. 4.18 Ureter and uterine vessels at the level of the middle part of the uterosacral ligaments. Right side. (1) Tube, (2) cul-de-sac of Douglas, (3) uterosacral ligament, (4) ureter, (5) internal iliac artery, (6) infundibulopelvic ligament, (7) obliterated umbilical artery

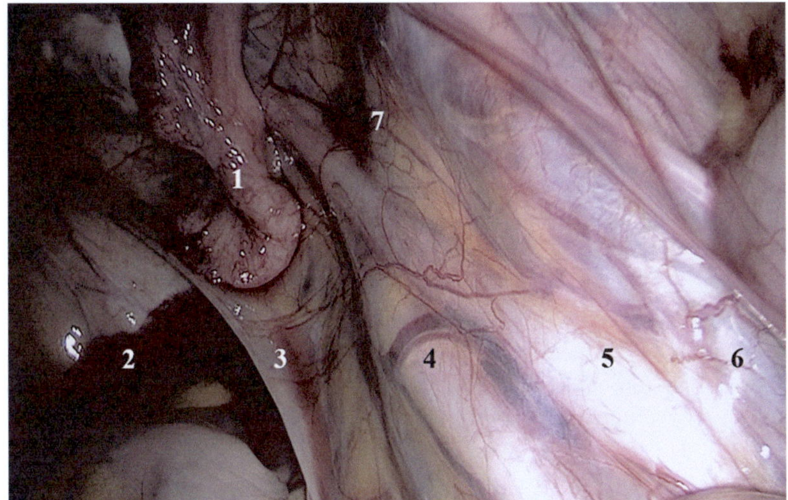

Fig. 4.19 Cohabitation with other pelvic structures. Right side. (1) Bowel, (2) tube and fimbria, (3) infundibulopelvic ligament, (4) external iliac artery, (5) ureter

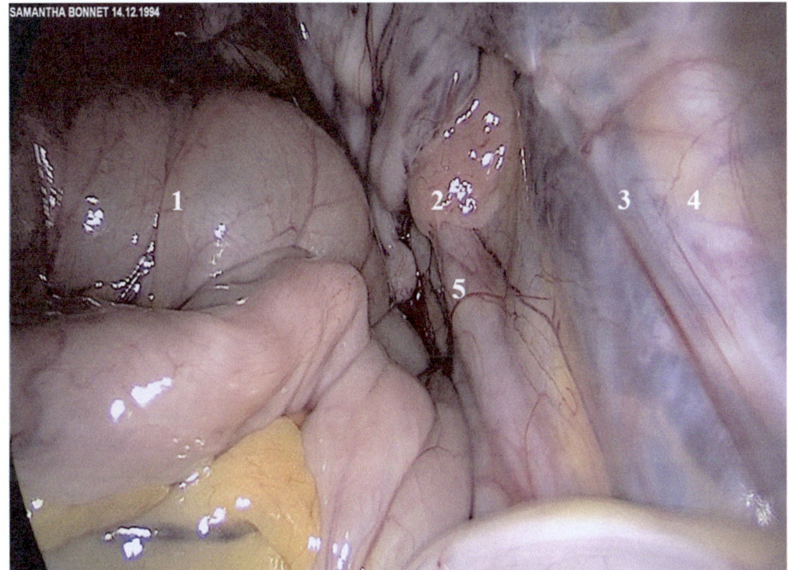

4.8 Ureter and Entry in the Mackenrodt's Ligament and into the Bladder (Figs. 4.20, 4.21 and 4.22)

Broad ligaments consist of loose areolar tissue wrapped by two layers of peritoneum. They connect the sides of the uterus to the lateral and posterior parts of the pelvis.

Just below, Mackenrodt's ligaments are weak fibroareolar that supports the uterus forming a fan-like structure spanning from the outside of the bladder to the outside of the sacrum. The two ligaments are situated over the endopelvic fascia, and the uterine veins lie below the fascia.

In a physiological situation, the proximity of the ureter and the vagina is evident (Fig. 4.20). Varicose uterine veins are sometimes visible, close to the lateral side of the uterus (Fig. 4.21).

The path of the ureter and its entry into the Mackenrodt's ligament (also called transverse or cardinal) can be seen by transparency through the peritoneum.

After vesicovaginal cleavage, the uterine artery is easy to identify and visualize (Fig. 4.22).

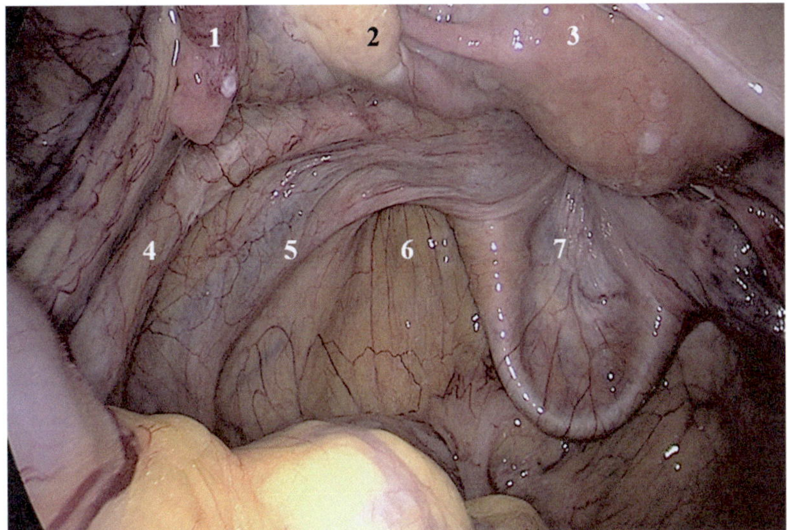

Fig. 4.20 Ureter before entry in the Mackenrodt's ligament. The vaginal retractor. Left side. (1) Fallopian tube, (2) ovary, (3) uterus, (4) ureter, (5) uterosacral ligament, (6) cul-de-sac of Douglas, (7) vaginal retractor placed in the posterior cul-de-sac of the vagina

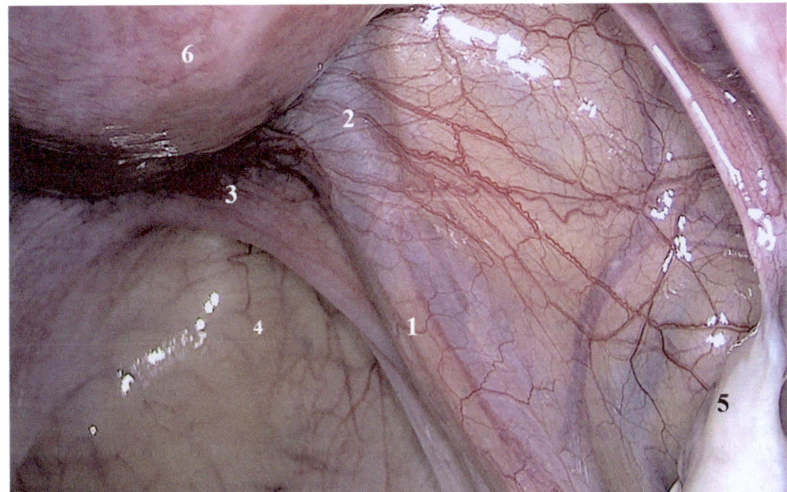

Fig. 4.21 Ureter before entry in the Mackenrodt's ligament. Venous uterine plexus. Right side. (1) Ureter, (2) uterine vessels, (3) uterosacral ligament, (4) cul-de-sac of Douglas, (5) ovary, (6) uterus

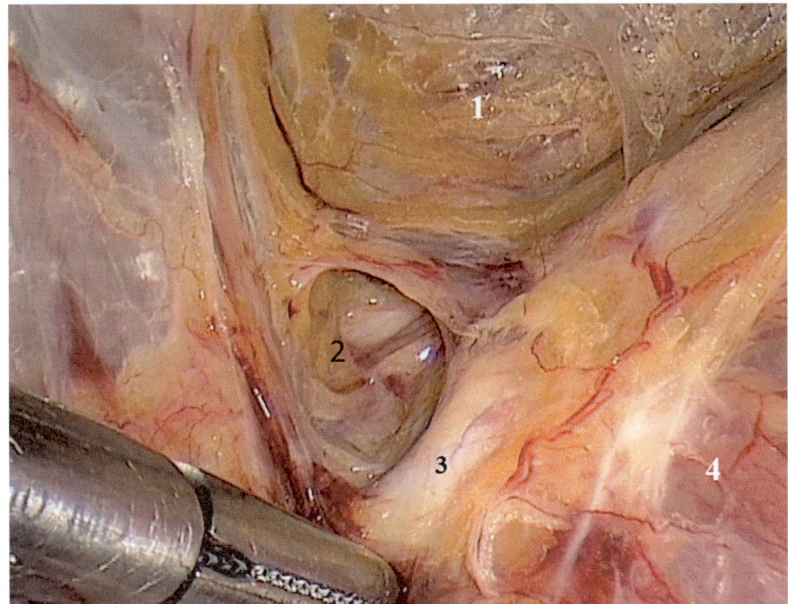

Fig. 4.22 Ureter before entry in the bladder. After vesicovaginal cleavage performed laterally. Vision of the ureter. Left side. (1) Bladder, (2) ureter, (3) uterine artery, (4) uterus

References

1. Kamina P. Anatomie clinique, deuxième édition, Tome 4. Maloine; 2008. p. 33–43.
2. Puntambekar S, Manchanda R. Surgical pelvic anatomy in gynecologic oncology. Int J Gynecol Obstet. 2018;143(52):86–92.

## Part II

Lesions of the Ureter in Surgical Gynecology

© The Author(s), under exclusive license to Springer Nature Switzerland AG 2022
J.-B. Dubuisson et al., *Ureteral Complications of Gynecological Surgery*,
https://doi.org/10.1007/978-3-031-15598-7_5

In Chap. 5, iatrogenic lesions of the ureter during pelvic surgery are described: thread ligatures, section, and compression by crushing, burn, adventitial stripping, and kink.

The traumatic lesions of the ureter are essentially secondary to urological, gynecological, and general surgery. About 90% of cases are located on the pelvic segment of the ureter [1]. In gynecology, only 33% of cases are identified intraoperatively. Stricture formation with complete obstruction leads to hydronephrotic atrophy of the kidney. Fistula formation may follow transection, crushing, or denudation injuries. The loss of continuity of the ureter manifests with an enclosed retroperitoneal urinoma or a urinary discharge from the operative site or the vagina.

Seven different types of ureteral injury are described.

5.1 Thread Ligature (Figs. 5.1, 5.2 and 5.3)

Thread ligatures are done usually during open surgery or vaginal surgery. Classically, it is seen in more than two-thirds of cases of ureteral injuries (Fig. 5.1).

Right after complete obstruction with a ligature, violent contractions of the ureter occur. After 1 h, the activity becomes intermittent and ceases, becoming a chronic obstruction. The loop that takes up the ureter causes a partial or complete obstruction with upstream stasis and renal deterioration. When there is an intraluminal pressure greater than glomerular filtration pressure, glomerular filtration decreases. If ureteral obstruction continues, hydronephrosis appears and causes nephron destruction within a few days. Even after adequate and quick treatment, the glomerular function recovers to some extent but rarely to completely normal levels.

Ligation is followed by ischemic necrosis with associated urine leakage in case of delayed management.

The first management to be considered is the section of the ligature, generally made easily by laparoscopy (Fig. 5.2).

If diagnosis and section of the ligation are made quite quickly in the 48 h following the injury, the ureter recovers well with the help of a ureteral stent (Fig. 5.3).

Fig. 5.1 Laparoscopic view of a thread ligature. Right side. The right ureter is included in a ligature, during a hysterectomy procedure. (1) Ureter and its course (yellow), (2) ligature

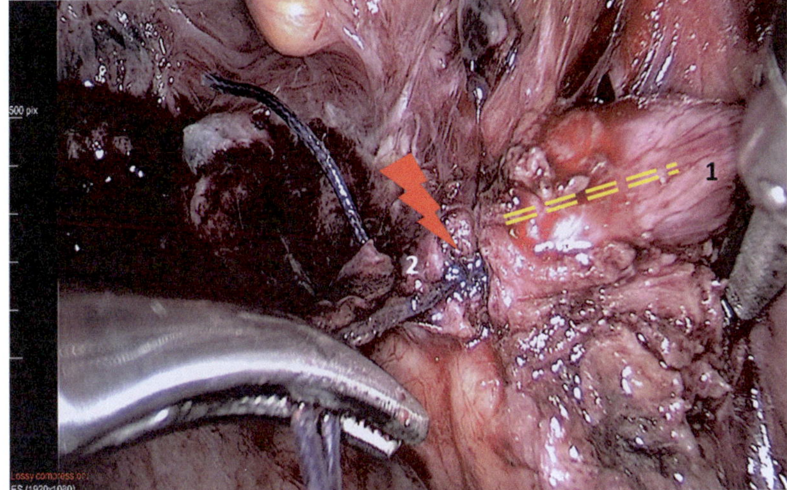

Fig. 5.2 Thread ligature. Section of the ligature obstructing the ureter. Right side. The loop that takes up the ureter is cut. (1) Ureter, (2) section of the suture

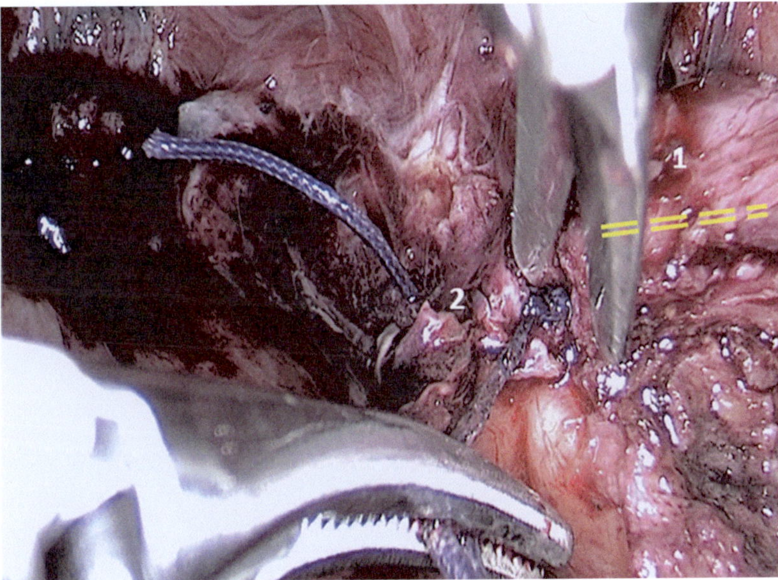

Fig. 5.3 Normal ureter after ligature section. Right side. Mobility and aspect are normal few minutes after the section of the suture. (1) Ureter, (2) Suture cut

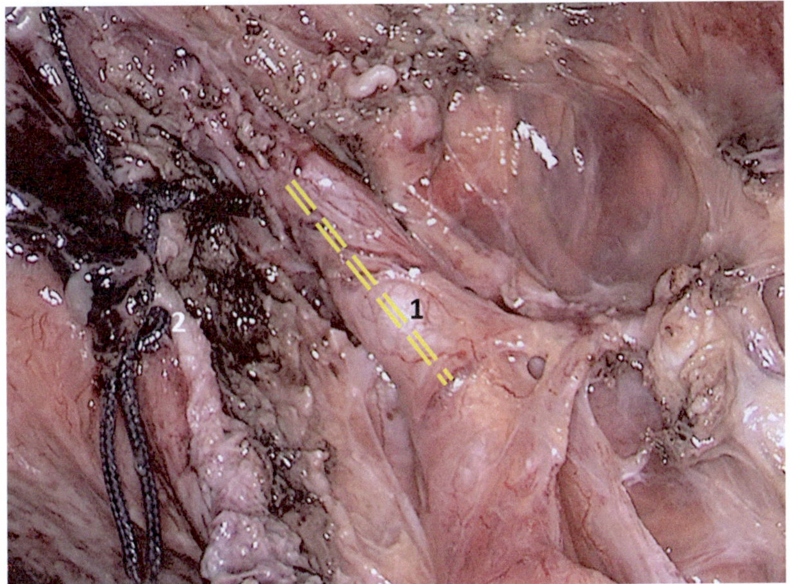

5.2 Section (Figs. 5.4, 5.5 and 5.6)

The ureter may be partially or entirely cut during hysterectomy, oophorectomy, or endometriosis excision (Fig. 5.4).

It may be lacerated during the dissection, for instance, in the case of deep infiltrating endometriosis, broad ligament leiomyoma, or ovarian tumor (Fig. 5.5).

The section of the ureter is quickly manifested by immediate urine leakage and fistulation (Fig. 5.6).

5.3 Compression by Crushing

The ureter may be crushed in a clamp. It will necrotize and then stricture at the site. A clamp placed too close to the ureter or a passage of a suture elbowing may have the same effect. This will cause stenosis but also may affect the blood supply. Devascularization should cause a secondary ureteral or ureterovaginal fistula.

Fig. 5.4 Intraoperative ureteral injury: complete section of the ureter. Right side. Section of the ureter during laparoscopic procedure. We see that the coagulations and section before reaching the uterine artery were too lateral and deep. (1) Level of the cup of the uterine manipulator, (2) right uterosacral ligament, (3) cul-de-sac of Douglas, (4) ovary, (5) round ligament

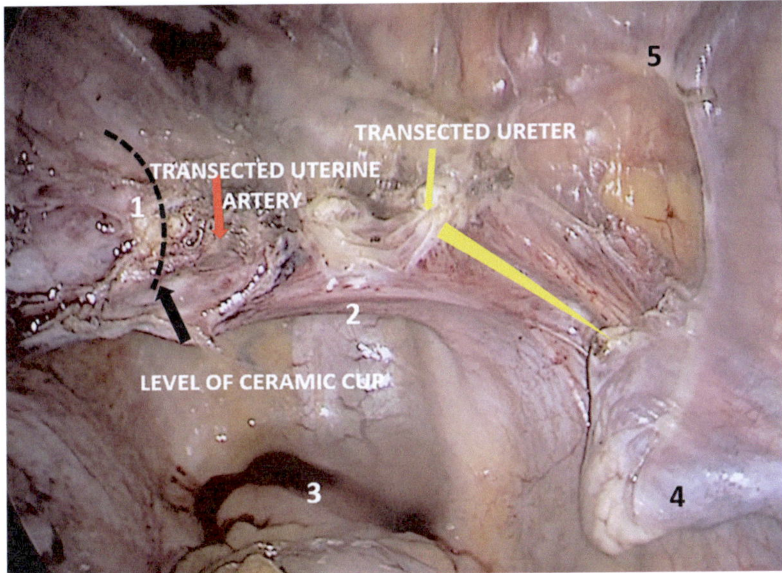

Fig. 5.5 Surgery for deep endometriosis. Section of the ureter during laparoscopic excision of endometriotic lesions. Right side. (1) Section of the ureter, (2) resected endometriotic lesions, (3) cul-de-sac of Douglas

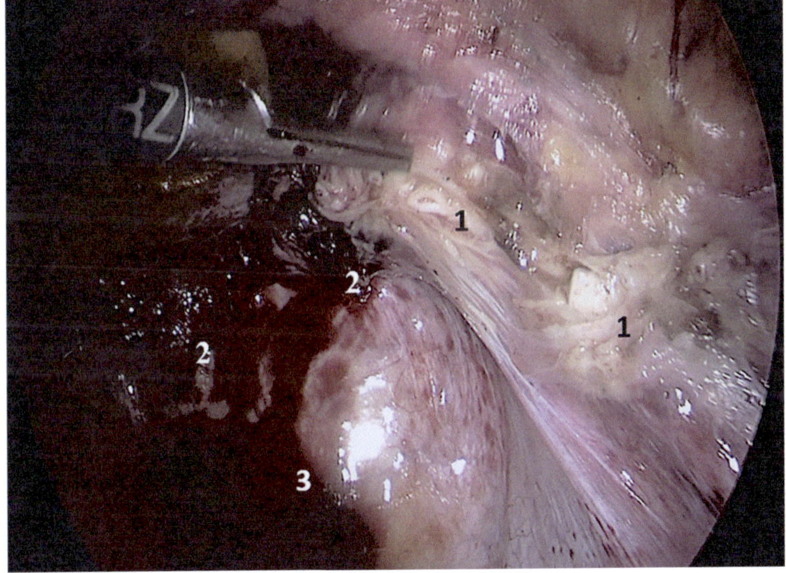

Fig. 5.6 Intraoperative ureteral injury: complete section of the ureter. Right side. Section after coagulation before its entry in the broad ligament. The section is different from a section of artery: no bleeding at the level of the section of ureter and urine leaks. (1) ureter, (2) uterosacral ligament

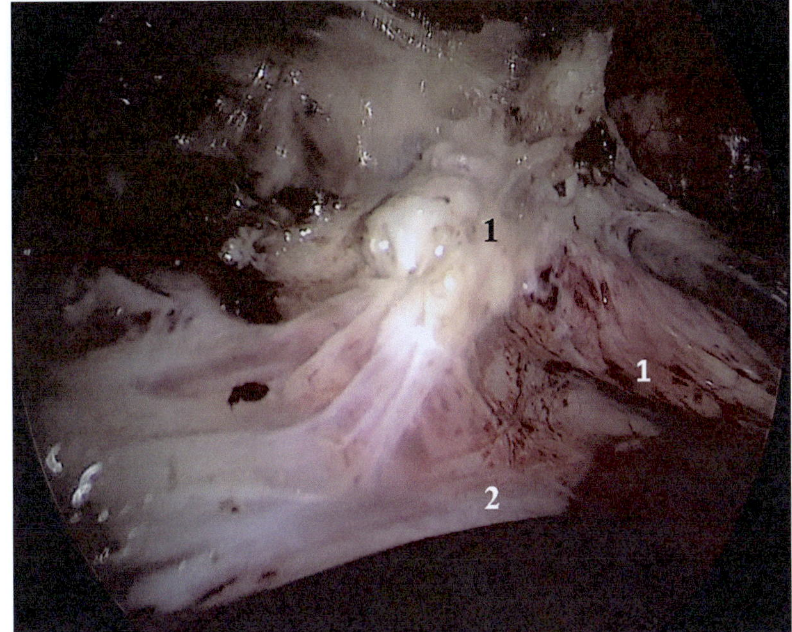

5.4 Burn and Diathermy-Related Injury (Fig. 5.7)

Burning of the ureter follows the secondary thermal diffusion by applying too close bipolar energy, ultrasound, or thermofusion with sealing of the vessels and tissue structures. Close to the forceps, the burn of the ureter often progresses to focal necrosis, then delayed fistula with uroperitoneum, urinoma, or vaginal leakage.

5.5 Denudation, Operative Adventitial Stripping

As the blood supply of the ureter is the adventitial coat, the stripping of this layer may cause necrosis at the site with changes resulting in stricture formation, stenosis, and fistula. It may be observed in the case of extended dissection of the lower ureter during radical surgery as Wertheim operation.

5.6 Perforation During an Endoluminal Procedure

It is mainly observed in urology.

5.7 Kink

The risk to kink the ureter mainly exists during pelvic prolapse surgery, including high uterosacral ligament suspension, performed by transvaginal access or by laparoscopy. The laparoscopic vision enables visualizing the course of the ureters, the symmetry of the suspension, and strongly decreases the risk of ureteral injury during the procedure. The vNOTES approach offers the same benefits in comparison to the conventional blinded transvaginal approach.

Another risk of kinking is during peritonealization of the mesh following sacrocolpopexy. This step concerns exclusively the right ureter.

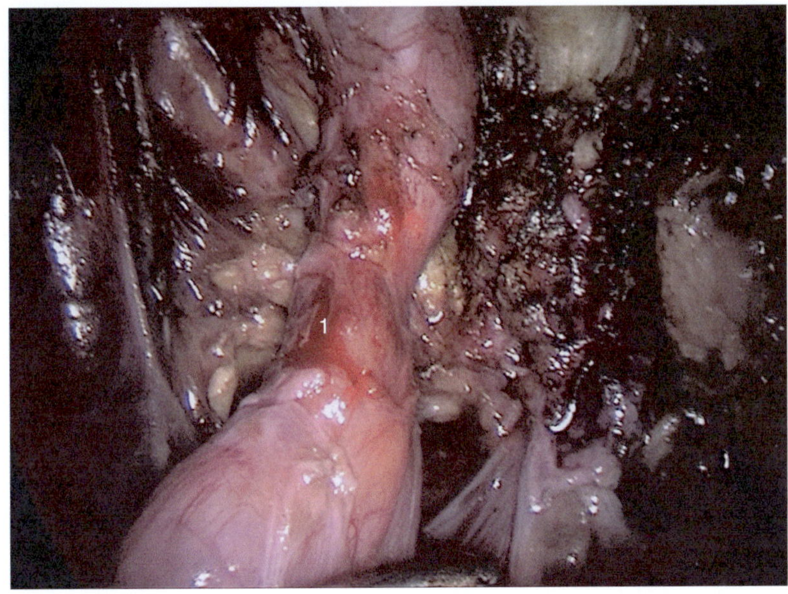

Fig. 5.7 Stenosis of the ureter after diathermy-related injury. Left side. The burn of the ureter progresses to fibrosis and stenosis. (1) Stenosis of the ureter

Reference

1. Selzman AA, Spirnak JP. Iatrogenic ureteral injuries: a 20-year experience in treating 165 injuries. J Urol. 1996;155(3):878–81.

Operations Causing Iatrogenic Lesions of the Ureter

6

© The Author(s), under exclusive license to Springer Nature Switzerland AG 2022
J.-B. Dubuisson et al., *Ureteral Complications of Gynecological Surgery*,
https://doi.org/10.1007/978-3-031-15598-7_6

Chapter 6 describes the main causes of iatrogenic injuries of the ureter in gynecological surgery: hysterectomy and its danger zones, oophorectomy, surgery for deep endometriosis, radical hysterectomy, genital prolapse, and stress urinary incontinence treatments. Injuries may be observed during obstetrical practice, meaning cesarean section and its hemorrhagic complications as well as postpartum hysterectomy.

Gynecological surgery is the main surgery responsible for injuries to the ureter, in over 50% of cases, with immediate recognition in a third of cases.

Ureteral complications may occur in 0.2–1.5% of gynecological operations.

6.1 Hysterectomy

Hysterectomy is performed in the great majority of cases for benign pathology such as leiomyoma and adenomyosis. In this circumstance, the occurrence of a severe ureteral complication is a major issue for the woman. Why? Because in many cases, the patient considers that this operation is rather easy and with a short recovery, according to the surgeon's explanations. 75% of ureteral injuries in gynecology are related to hysterectomy procedures.

6.1.1 Danger Zones

The danger zones of injury of the ureter are well defined.

6.1.1.1 Crossing of the Iliac Vessels (Fig. 6.1)

The crossing of the iliac vessels and the close insertion of the infundibulopelvic ligament into the ovary concerns about 25% of cases. It is observed during associated oophorectomy, difficult lysis of the adnexa, or large ovarian tumors. This localization is well explained on the left side due to the presence of the sigmoid colon and its meso, often associated with a fatty envelope.

At this level, on the right and left sides, severe adhesions (endometriosis, postoperative condition), large tumors, or obesity may explain this complication.

Fig. 6.1 Place of danger during hysterectomy: crossing of the iliac vessels. Right side. (1) Iliac vessels, (2) ureter, (3) infundibulopelvic ligament, (4) ovary, (5) cul-de-sac of Douglas

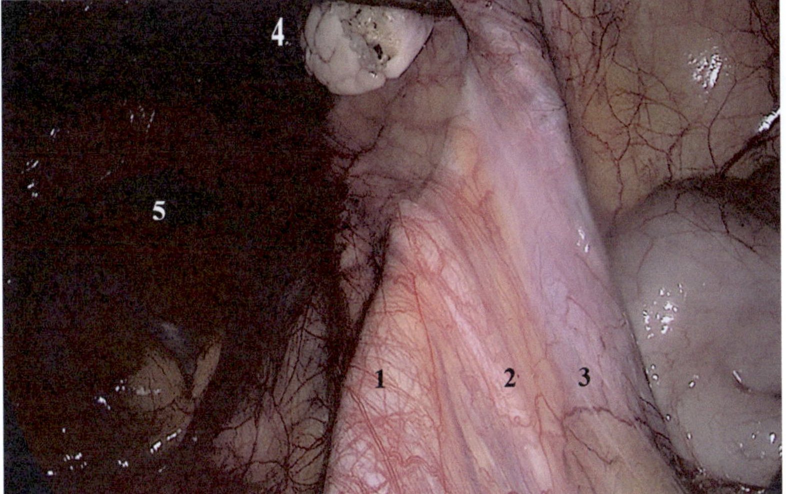

6.1.1.2 Crossing of the Uterine Arteries
(Figs. 6.2 and 6.3)

The crossing of the uterine artery is the most relevant danger zone. This is in relation to the hysterectomy procedure, a common operation in gynecology. During this procedure, hemostasis and a section of the uterine pedicle are performed at the level of the internal opening of the cervix. There is usually a 2 cm distance between the cervix and the ureter, but this distance could vary. A distance of only 0.5 cm can be observed in 3% of women with normal anatomy. This area concerns about 50% of ureteral injuries (Fig. 6.2).

Ureteral injury is mainly observed during total hysterectomy, and more rarely during supracervical hysterectomy. The technique of pulling up the uterus during open and laparoscopic hysterectomy distances from the ureter is to prevent this kind of complication. At the crossing of the uterine artery, at the level of the internal orifice of the cervix, the risk of the accident remains low but increases when the operative field is bloody, caused by poor vessel hemostasis. In this difficult condition, the surgeon may have an insufficient vision, leading to the injury of the ureter or its surrounding tissue (Fig. 6.3).

The ureter may also be injured at its entry into the bladder, especially occurring during radical hysterectomy.

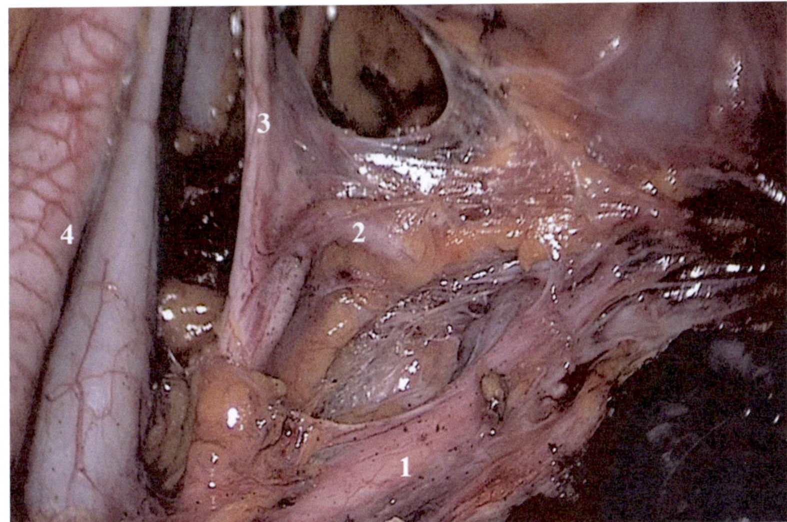

Fig. 6.2 Place of danger of ureter injury: bifurcation of the umbilical artery and uterine artery and crossing of the uterine arteries. Left side. Laparoscopic view. Retroperitoneal dissection. (1) Ureter, (2) uterine artery at its origin, (3) obliterated umbilical artery (medial umbilical ligament), (4) Iliac vessels dissected

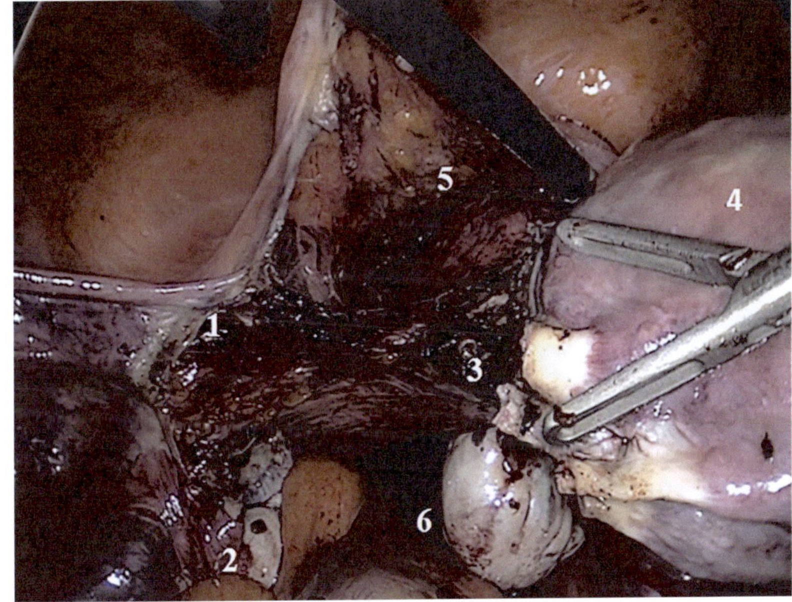

Fig. 6.3 Place of danger of ureteral injury: crossing and after crossing during total laparoscopic hysterectomy. Coagulation and section in the ascending portion of the uterine artery, done above the crossing. Left side. The left ureter in not visible, below the area of the uterine artery. (1) Round ligament, (2) Adnexa, (3) Uterine artery transsected, (4) Uterus, (5) Bladder (lift), (6) Right ovary

6.1.1.3 Colpotomy (Figs. 6.4 and 6.5)

Ureteral injury during the section of the vagina (colpotomy) is uncommon. In normal conditions, the colpotomy is performed far from the ureter, thus avoiding any thermal damage during hemostasis. The risk is higher in the case of injuries to vessels, provoking a severe hemorrhage and difficult hemostasis. The bad vision of the field and the excessive use of energy explain the complication (Fig. 6.4).

Through laparoscopy, magnification of the laparoscope helps to perform the colpotomy at the precise site between the cervix and vagina (Fig. 6.5).

Fig. 6.4 Places of danger of ureter injury during hysterectomy: colpotomy. Section of the vagina using the uterine manipulator. (1) Manipulator cup, (2) vagina, (3) uterine vessels transsected, (4) uterus isthmus

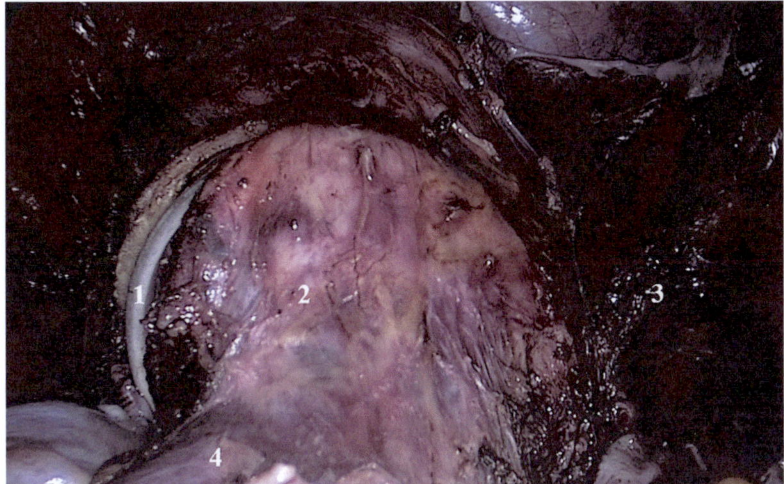

Fig. 6.5 Places of danger of ureter injury during total laparoscopic hysterectomy: colpotomy. Right side. (1) Cervix, (2) Cup of the uterine manipulator, (3) Transsected uterine vessels, (4) Uterosacral ligament

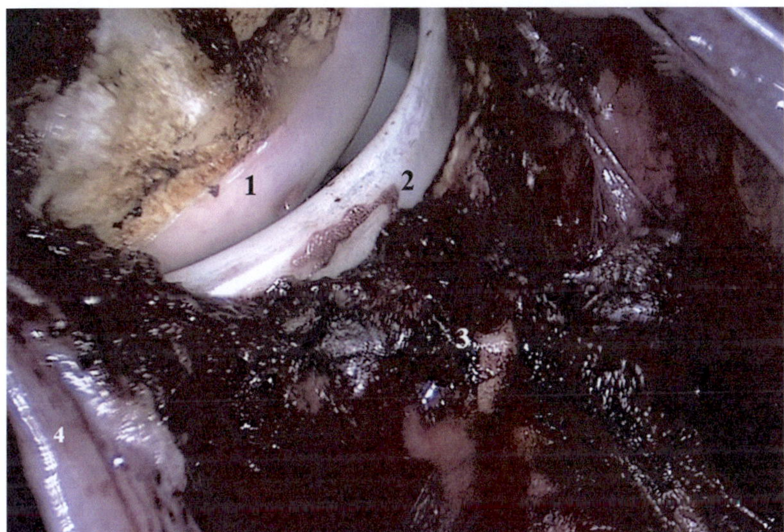

6.1.1.4 Closure of the Vagina and Fascia (Figs. 6.6, 6.7 and 6.8)

The risk of ureteral injury is observed at the lateral angles if the suture is too deep, in general, if the hemostasis of branches of the vaginal arteries is difficult (Fig. 6.6).

The ureteral check at the end of the procedure is mandatory, including the visualization of the ureter after the vaginal cuff closure, its distance, and integrity (caliber and peristalsis) (Figs. 6.7 and 6.8).

The other danger zones are less frequent, in the broad ligament, or during the uncrossing, in approximately 25% of cases, and very rarely during peritonealization after hysterectomy (ureteral kink).

Precise inspection of the pelvis and the entire abdomen before starting any surgical procedure is needed. For instance, rare anomalies may be seen: the pelvic kidney, ureteral duplication, and kidney agenesia. The pelvic kidney is the most frequent: it is due to a failure to ascend to a normal position in the upper abdomen. The kidney is located inferior to the promontory, and the ureters are shorter than normal. An injury of the ureter during its abnormal course is possible.

Incidence Rate During Hysterectomy

The rate of ureteral injury is classically 2.5% of hysterectomies, 2% after radical hysterectomy, and postoperative radiotherapy [1]. The evaluation has been done more recently after laparoscopic hysterectomy [2–4]. Harkki-Siren et al. [2] observed 13.9 per 1000 ureteral lesions. Chapron et al. [4] observed 2.5% of major urinary complications with 1 in 313 patients of the ureteral lesion, 0.35% after total hysterectomy. In a review of English language publications for the past 10 years, by Adelman et al. [5], the overall urinary tract injury rate for laparoscopic hysterectomy was 0.73%. They note a rate of ureteric complications of between 0.02% and 0.4%. But the undetected lesions are more frequent according to studies when performing an intraoperative cystoscopy with an injection of carmine indigo [6].

In the large series by Kiran et al. [7], from 2001 to 2010, 377,073 women had a hysterectomy, among which 1792 (0.5%) presented a ureteral injury. After 2006, ureteral lesions were more frequent in abdominal radical hysterectomy for uterine cancer (10.7%) than in hysterectomy for benign pathology (less than 1%). However, patients who had a hysterectomy associated with endometriosis presented a ureteral lesion in 1.7% of cases, which is, therefore, more frequent. As for uterine cancer, Li et al. [8] report a ureteral obstruction rate of 2.18% after radical hysterectomy and postoperative radiotherapy.

In another publication, Hesselman et al. [9] studied a longitudinal population-based register study of 25,354 women who had a benign hysterectomy at 46 hospital units in Sweden between 2000 and 2014. This study confirmed that endometriosis increased the risk of ureter injury (adjusted odds ratio, 2.15; 95% confidence interval, 1.34–3.44).

In a recent publication, Chang et al. [10] published a retrospective population-based observational study concerning 501,110 women who had undergone hysterectomy for benign pathology between 2012 and 2015. They included as follows total abdominal hysterectomy (56.7%), total laparoscopic hysterectomy (12.1%), abdominal supracervical hysterectomy (11.1%), laparoscopic-assisted vaginal hysterectomy (9.1%), total vaginal hysterectomy (7%), and laparoscopic supracervical hysterectomy (4%). They noted that vesicoureteral injury was reported in 0.21% of cases overall. Total laparoscopic hysterectomy (0.13%) had the highest ureteral injury rate, whereas total abdominal hysterectomy had the lowest (0.04%). The risk of ureteral injury was particularly high when a total laparoscopic hysterectomy was performed for endometriosis (OR 6.15, 95% CI 1.18–31.9, $p = 0.031$) or uterine leiomyoma (OR 4.15, 95% CI 2.13–8.11, $p < 0.001$).

Fig. 6.6 Prevention of ureteric injury: Closure of the vaginal vault during total laparoscopic hysterectomy. Right side. (1) Bladder, (2) colpotomy (vaginal wall), (3) uterus removed and placed in the vagina to avoid the CO_2 leak

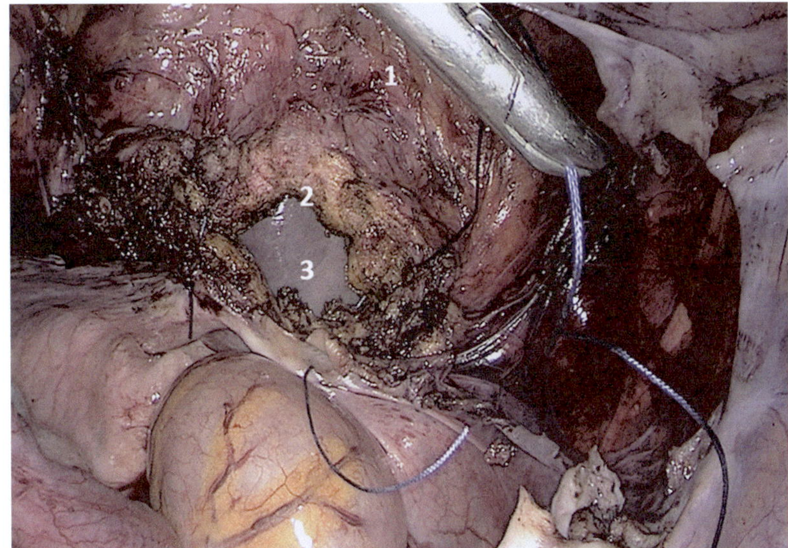

Fig. 6.7 Traumatic injuries of the ureter. Vaginal vault closure after total hysterectomy. The panoramic view shows that the suture is normally far from the ureters going to the depth of the Mackenrodt's ligaments. (1) Bladder, (2) vaginal cuff closure, (3) uterine vessels coagulated, (4) left uterosacral ligament

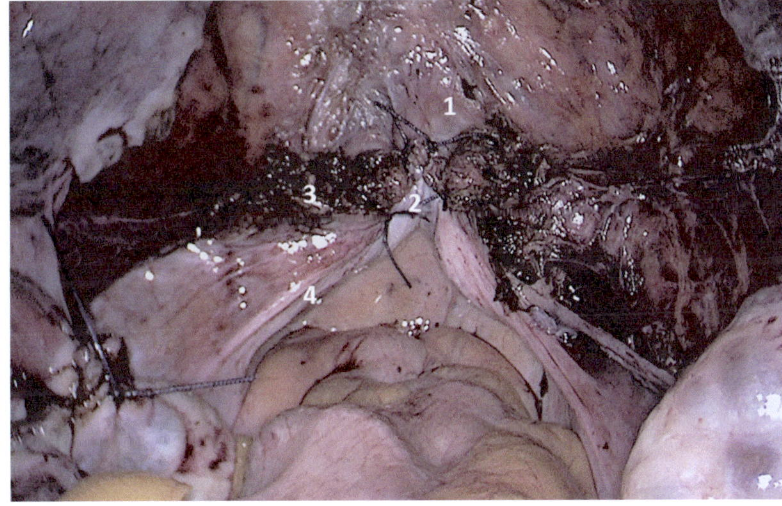

Fig. 6.8 Traumatic injuries of the ureter. The control at the end of total laparoscopic hysterectomy: situation of the ureter in relation to the scar of the vaginal vault after total hysterectomy. Right side. (1) Bladder, (2) vaginal cuff closed, (3) cul-de-sac of Douglas, (4) right uterosacral ligament, (5) ureter (caliber and peristalsis)

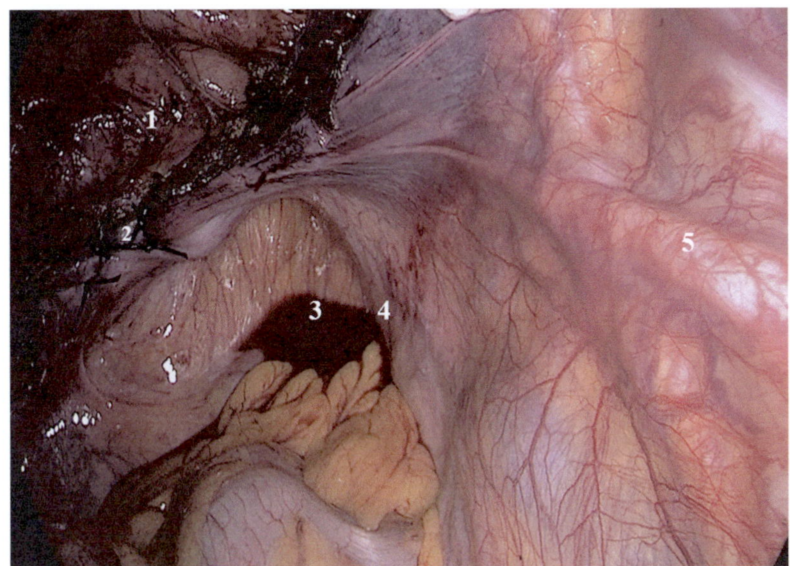

6.2 Hysterectomy Associated with Adnexal Surgery and Ovariolysis (Figs. 6.9, 6.10 and 6.11)

In the case of adnexectomy, the ureter may be injured at the level of the infundibulopelvic ligament or the ovarian fossa. It is quite rare in the absence of adhesions and with the use of bipolar coagulation because of the sufficient distance between the two structures (Fig. 6.9).

In case of severe adhesions, organs are stuck to each other making the ovariolysis more difficult and more hazardous. Different techniques exist to visualize and individualize the infundibulopelvic ligament. The easiest technique is lateral pelvic dissection (Fig. 6.10). The incision of the peritoneum is made laterally, external to the adnexa in the area of the pelvic triangle. The retroperitoneal dissection in this "healthy area" facilitates the visualization of the ureter, the uterine artery, and the infundibulopelvic ligament. Then the operative procedure is performed with a maximum of safety (Fig. 6.11).

Fig. 6.9 Laparoscopic hysterectomy associated with oophorectomy with visualization of the ureter. Right side. (1) Bowel, (2) uterosacral ligament, (3) ureter, (4) right infundibulopelvic ligament transsected, (5) posterior leaf of the broad ligament

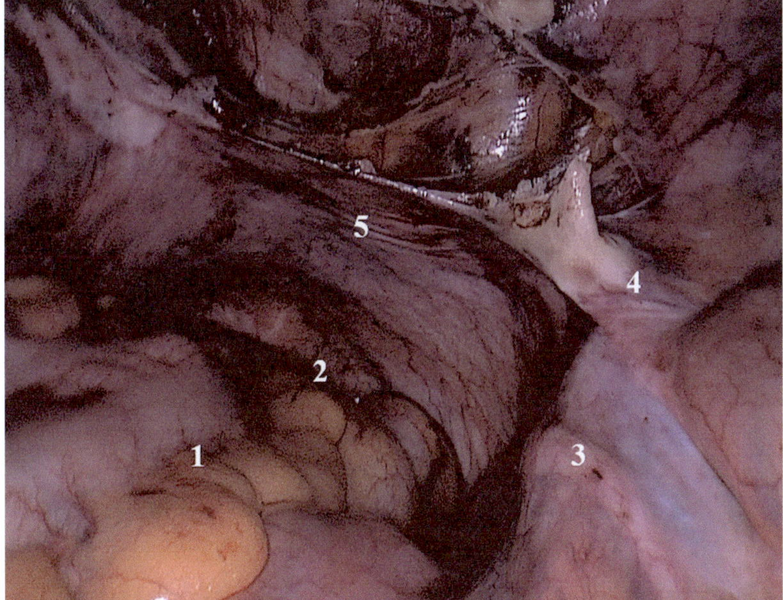

Fig. 6.10 Hysterectomy associated with surgery of adnexa and ovariolysis. Lateral pelvic lysis of the adnexa covered with cohesive adhesions. Severe adhesions sticking the organs together, making the ovariolysis more difficult and more dangerous. Right side. Laparoscopic view. (1) Medial part of the right ovary, (2) tube, (3) incision of the peritoneum lateral to the infundibulo-pelvic ligament to facilitate the visualization of the external iliac artery and after dissection, the ureter and the uterine artery, (4) bowel, (5) round ligament

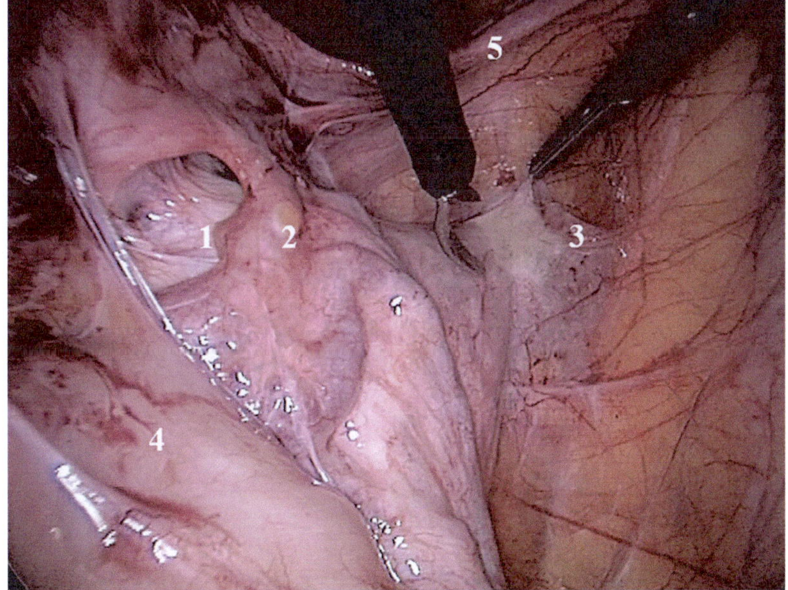

Fig. 6.11 Ureteric injuries and hysterectomy associated with surgery of the adnexa: Final laparosocpic view of the ureter after retroperitoneal dissection. Right side. (1) Ureter, (2) obliterated umbilical artery, (3) ovary

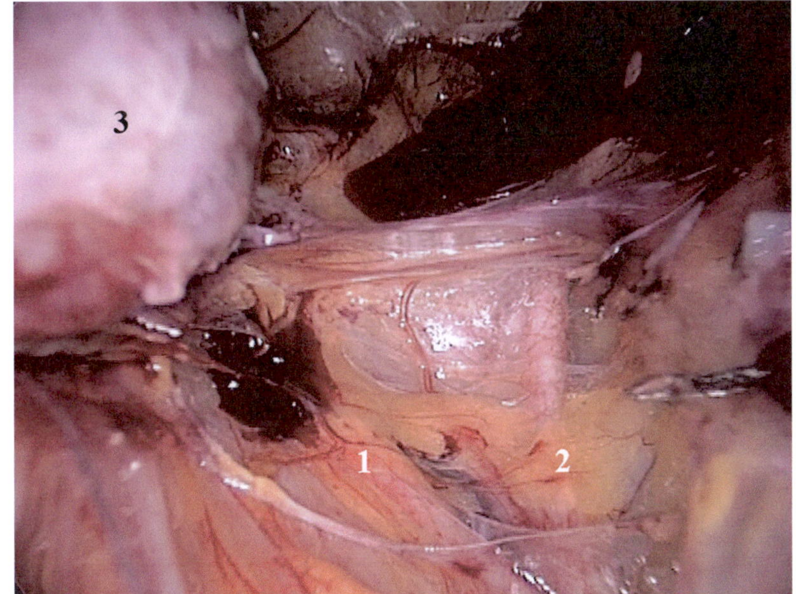

6.3   Oophorectomy (Figs. 6.12, 6.13 and 6.14)

The laparoscopic technique is described. Injury of the ureter can occur during oophorectomy, especially in difficult cases of ovarian malignancy, peritoneal carcinosis, or severe endometriosis. It is observed during coagulation-section and severing of the ovarian pedicle (Fig. 6.12).

It is mandatory to visualize the ureter before the section of the infundibulopelvic ligament.

The final step of the oophorectomy is the coagulation and section of the fallopian tube and the ovarian ligament, close to the uterine cornua (Fig. 6.13).

The final check of the ureter (caliber and peristalsis) after oophorectomy is recommended (Fig. 6.14).

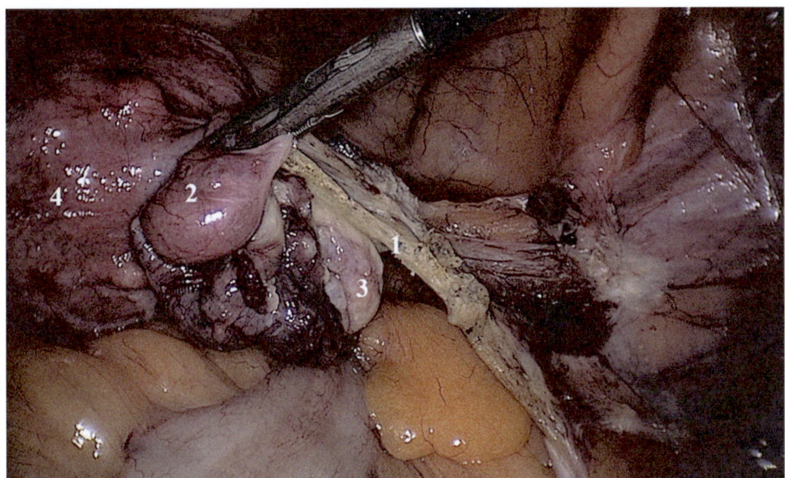

Fig. 6.12 Ureteric injuries and oophorectomy. Laparoscopic technique. Coagulation and section of the ovarian pedicle usually far from the ureter. Right side. (1) Site of oophorectomy, (2) fallopian tube, (3) ovary, (4) uterus

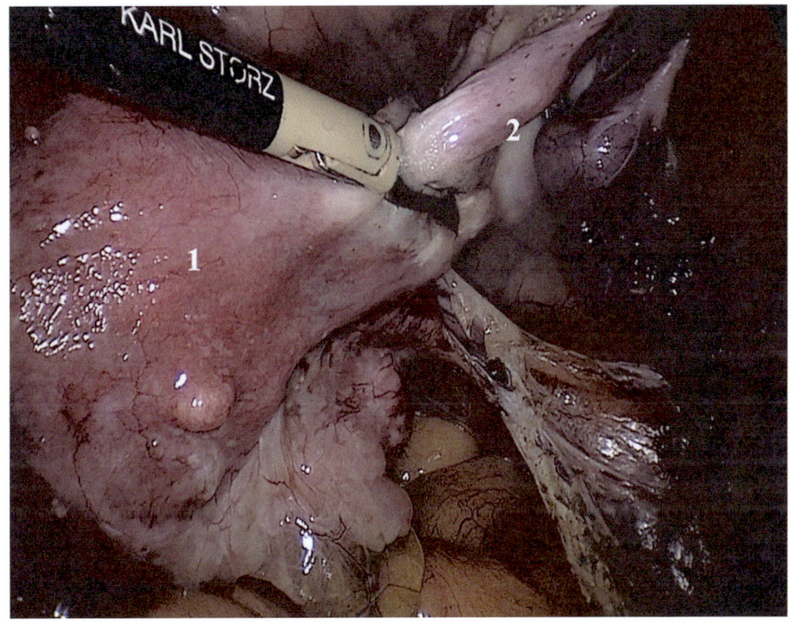

Fig. 6.13 Ureteric injuries and oophorectomy: End of procedure of laparoscopic oophorectomy with coagulation and section close to the cornua. Right side. (1) Uterus, (2) fallopian tube

Fig. 6.14 Ureteric injuries and oophorectomy. Control of the broad ligament after ovariolysis and oophorectomy, at a good distance from the ureter. Right side. Laparoscopic view. (1) Round ligament, (2) transsected infundibulopelvic ligament, (3) uterine cornua, (4) ureter, (5) uterosacral ligament, (6) cul-de-sac of Douglas

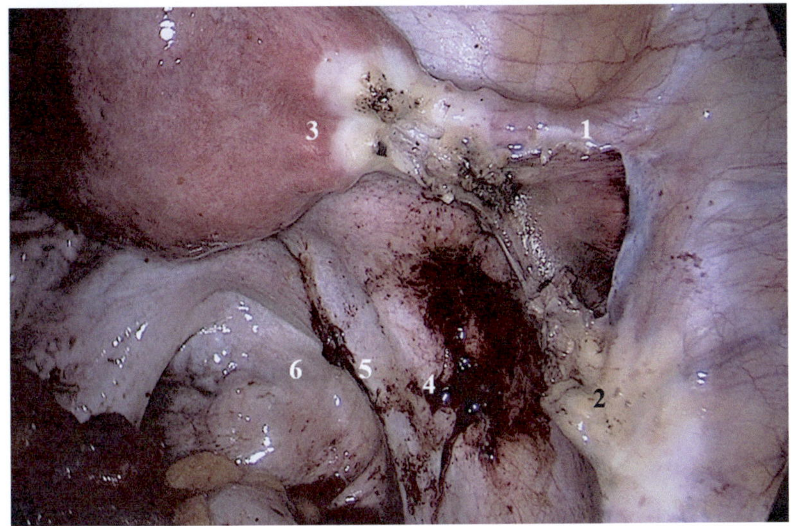

6.4　Surgery for Deep Endometriosis (Fig. 6.15)

The injury of the ureter may be observed in every case of pelvic endometriosis, especially with severe adhesions between ovaries, uterosacral ligaments, bowel, sigmoid colon, and rectum. It is observed during the excision of the endometriotic lesions.

6.4.1　Frozen Pelvis

In the case of the frozen pelvis, adhesions are severely upsetting the usual anatomical landmarks. The difficulty affects most of the time both the ureter and the intestine.

The section of the ureter may occur during extensive dissection of lateral lesions or posterior deep endometriotic nodules.

Fig. 6.15 Surgery of endometriosis. Risk of ureteral injury during excision of the endometriotic lesions. Cul-de-sac obliteration. Laparoscopic view. (1) Uterosacral ligament, (2) rectosigmoid adhesions, (3) uterus, (4) left ovary, (5) left tube, (6) endometriosis lesions with adhesions

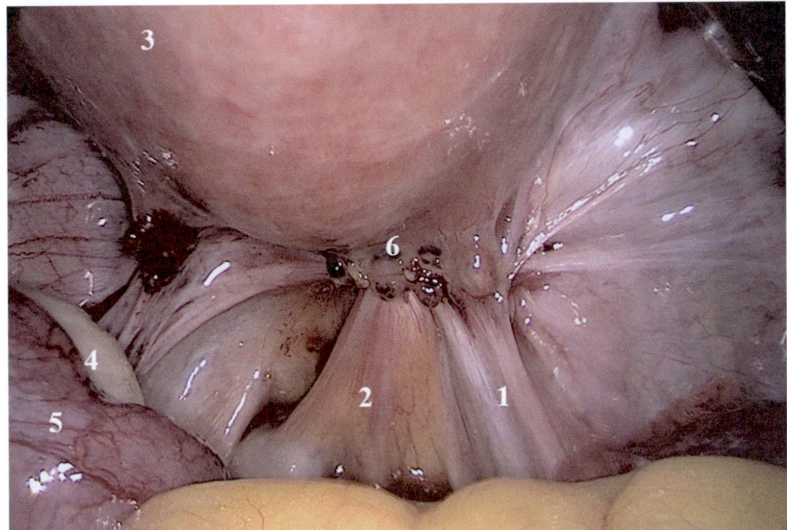

6.4.2 Severe Ovariolysis (Figs. 6.16 and 6.17)

In case of endometriosis and adhesions between the ovary and the ovarian fossa, the dissection is gently performed using atraumatic forceps (Fig. 6.16).

In the case of cohesive adhesions with welding of the ovary to the ovarian fossa, the dissection of the ovary is difficult, and often hemorrhagic (Fig. 6.17).

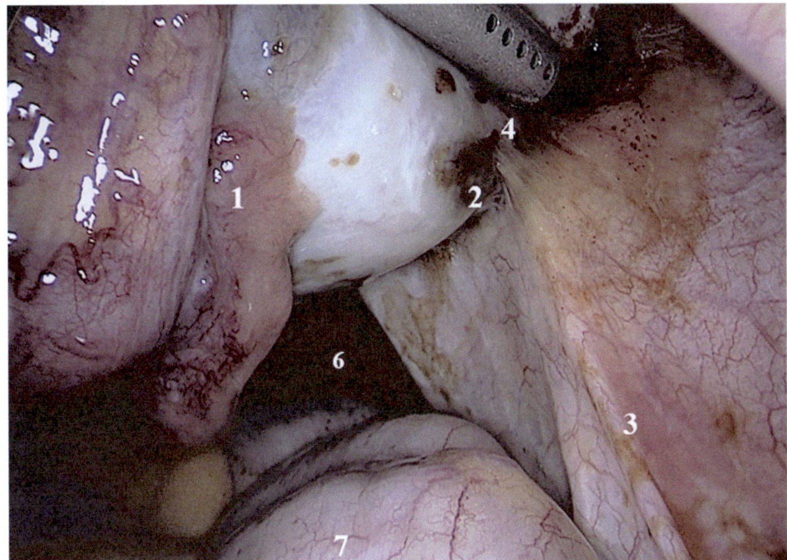

Fig. 6.16 Ureteric injury and ovariolysis. Gentle laparoscopic ovariolysis between ovary and ovarian fossa. Right side. The dissection may damage the ureter. (1) Fallopian tube, (2) fixed ovary, (3) ureter, (4) Ovarian fossa with beginning of cleavage using an atraumatic instrument, (5) infundibulopelvic ligament, (6) cul-de-sac of Douglas, (7) bowel

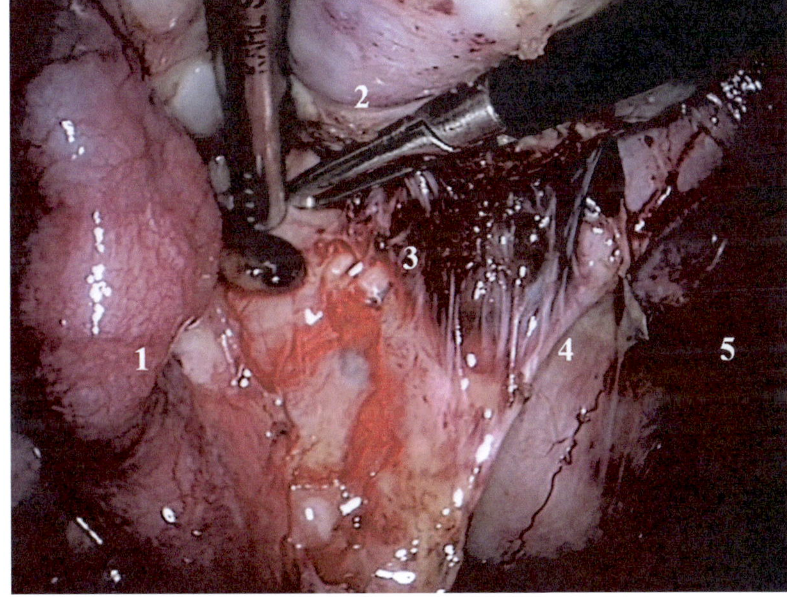

Fig. 6.17 Severe ovariolysis. Deep and peritoneal active endometriosis. Extensive welding of the ovary with the ovarian fossa and ureter. Left side. (1) Fallopian tube, (2) ovary, (3) severe adhesions between ovary and ovarian fossa, (4) uterosacral ligament, (5) cul-de-sac of Douglas

6.4.3 Heat Transmission (Fig. 6.18)

A heat transmission burn may occur around electrocoagulation or laser vaporization during extensive surgery near the ureter. Postoperatively, there is always a possibility of secondary stenosis during healing in the broad ligament and a risk of recurrence by direct invasion by the endometriotic process [11].

6.5 Radical Hysterectomy (Figs. 6.19, 6.20 and 6.21)

Specificities of radical hysterectomy are first to treat the uterine artery at its origin, with a large dissection of the paravesical and pararectal spaces; second to unroof the ureter in the parametrium.

The uterine artery originates from a trunk including the obliterated umbilical artery or directly from the anterior trunk of the internal iliac artery but several other variations exist.

The first step of the procedure consists of the transection of the uterine artery and the superficial uterine vein that runs together at the level of the internal iliac artery. Then the ureter is freed by blunt dissection till its entry into the parametrium. At this step, the bladder needs to be dissected, reaching the plane of the vesicovaginal septum, without treating the vesicouterine ligaments (Fig. 6.19).

The next step is to perform the ureteral tunnel, progressively separating the ureter from the surrounding parametrial tissue. Unroofing the ureter continues from the medial part of the anterior parametrium, along the adventitial sheath, gently lowering and lateralizing the ureter. "T" ureteric artery is inconstant at this level and can be clipped at this step. Then, the ureter is step by step separated from the parametrium. With opposite traction of the uterus and the bladder, the vesicouterine ligament is well exposed, enabling it to transect away from the prevesical visceral segment of the ureter. The ureter is followed till its entry into the bladder (Fig. 6.20).

The end of the procedure is the treatment itself of the lateral parametrium, the extension depending on the oncologic disease. The ureter is lateralized during the section of the parametrium (Fig. 6.21).

Fig. 6.18 Heat transmission. Deep and peritoneal endometriosis. Extensive excision of the endometriotic lesions developed in all the area of the posterior compartment. With this dissection, the risk of thermal injury of the ureter exists. (1) Uterus, (2) right tube, (3) left tube, (4) left ovary, (5) bowel, (6) area of excision of endometriosis with coagulation

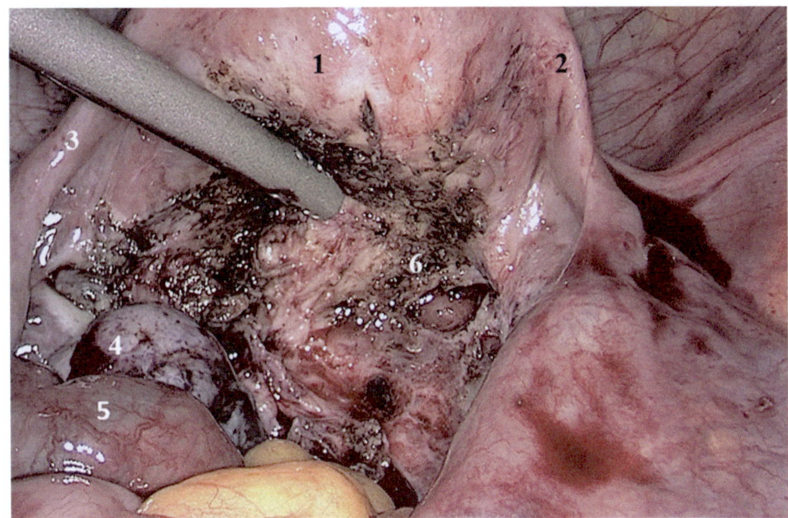

Fig. 6.19 Radical hysterectomy. Ventral parametrium. Left side. Laparoscopic view during radical hysterectomy. Red arrow indicates the way to unroof the ureter. (1) Ureter (clip on the "T" ureteric artery), (2) uterine artery transsected and lift, (3) vagina (vesicovaginal space), (4) vesicouterine ligament, (5) medial paravesical space

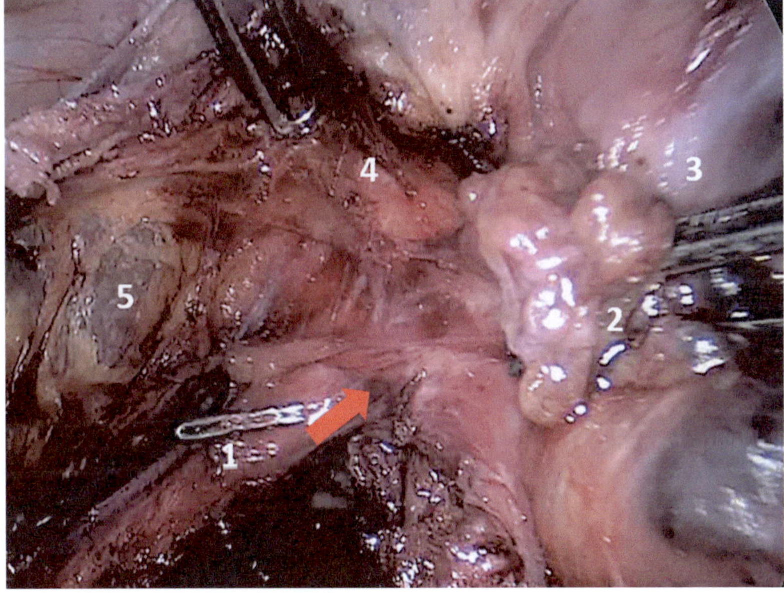

Fig. 6.20 Radical hysterectomy. Unroofed ureter. Left side. Laparoscopic view during radical hysterectomy. Uterus still in place. (1) Ureter totally freed, (2) transsected uterine pedicle, (3) bladder, (4) vagina

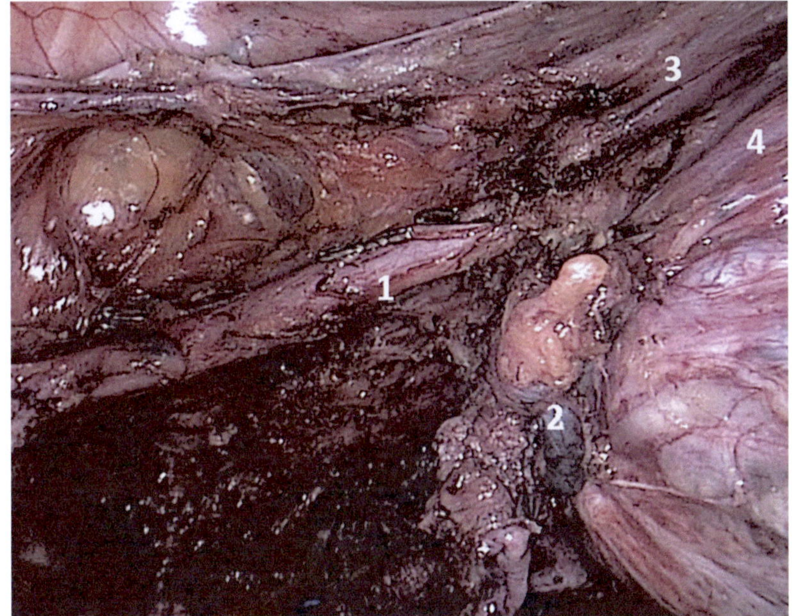

Fig. 6.21 Radical hysterectomy. Final view of the unroofed ureter after removal of the uterus. Right side. Laparoscopic view during radical hysterectomy. (1) Ureter, (2) vaginal cuff, (3) rectum, (4) bladder

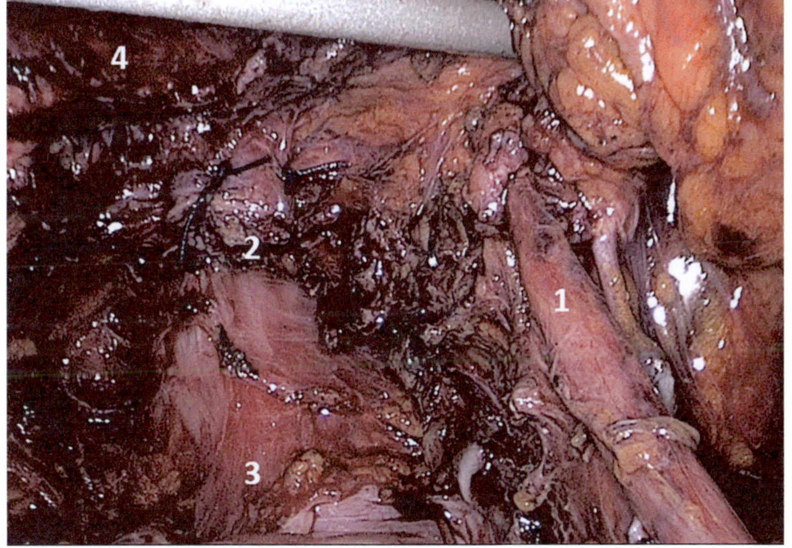

6.6 Vaginal Radical Hysterectomy (Schauta's Operation) (Figs. 6.22 and 6.23)

Initial surgical steps are the same for radical hysterectomy and trachelectomy. The difficulty of the procedure is the recognition of the ureter through the vaginal approach and its dissection to treat the parametrium with the same radicality as in the open or laparoscopic route.

The vaginal step is the mobilization of a 2 cm cuff of the vagina to cover the cervix. The vesicovaginal septum is entered and the paravesical space dissected. The ureter should be palpated at this level, thus enabling the division of the vesicouterine ligament (Fig. 6.22).

After the cutting of the vesicouterine ligament, the ureter at its distal segment ("knee") is pushed away to safely treat the lateral anterior and lateral parametrium (Fig. 6.23).

6.7 Perforation of the Isthmus of the Uterus

Occurring during dilatation and curettage or hysteroscopy, uterine perforation can be complicated by damage to the uterine vessels and the ureter. This kind of complication is very rare.

Fig. 6.22 Vaginal radical hysterectomy. Paravesical space entered. Left side. Left ureter is palpated with the "rolling" finger. (1) Paravesical space, (2) vesicocaginal septum, (3) vaginal cuff covering the cervix

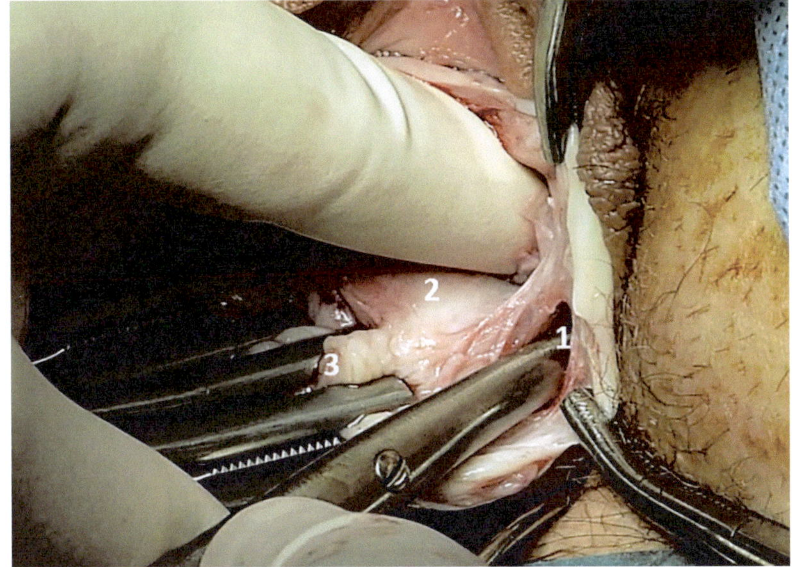

Fig. 6.23 Vaginal radical hysterectomy. Ureteral dissection at the "knee" level (distal segment) after section of the vesicouterine ligament. Left side. (1) Ureter, (2) vesicovagial space, (3) paravesical space, (4) cervix covered by the vaginal cuff

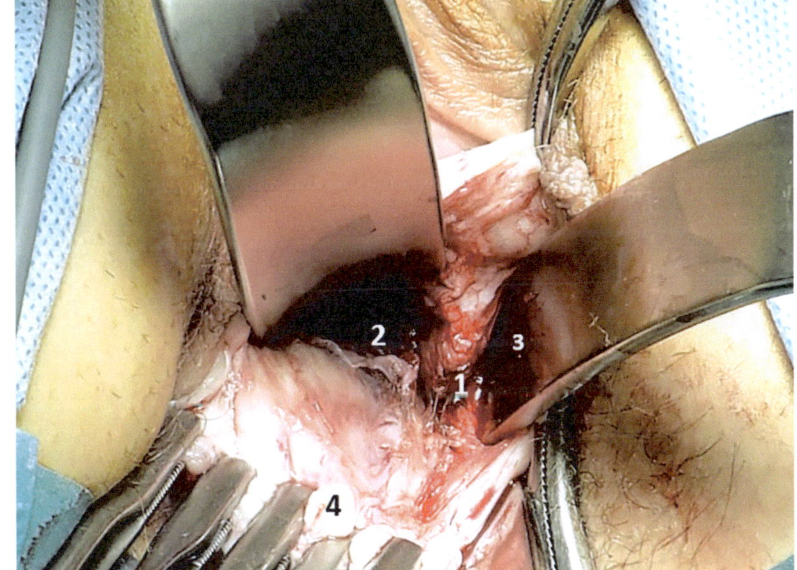

6.8 Pelvic Organ Prolapse
(Figs.6.24, 6.25, 6.26 and 6.27)

During surgery for pelvic organ prolapse, including mainly high suspension of the uterosacral ligaments, the ureter can be taken from the upper plications of the uterosacral ligaments made vaginally or laparoscopically (Fig. 6.24).

Vaginally, it can also be kinked during an anterior colporrhaphy with vaginal fascia plications in case of severe prolapse, due to the descending course of the ureter in this condition (Fig. 6.25).

The risk of injury during laparoscopic treatment of pelvic organ prolapse is low (Fig. 6.26). Usually, the dissections for plications or fixation of meshes are performed in the central part of the pelvis, for example, vesicovaginal cleavage or rectovaginal cleavage. Considering the sacrocolpopexy, the risk of ureteral injury concerns the dissection of the anterior longitudinal ligament at the level of the promontory.

During vesicovaginal cleavage, there is no need to dissect too laterally. When the dissection goes too laterally, the risk of injury to the ureter exists, aggravated by distortion of the organs caused by prolapse (Fig. 6.27).

Fig. 6.24 Causes of ureteric injury. Surgery for pelvic organ prolapse. Laparoscopic high plications of the uterosacral ligaments. (1) Plications of uterosacral ligaments, (2) right ureter in this area, (3) right ovary, (4) cul-de-sac of Douglas, (5) uterus

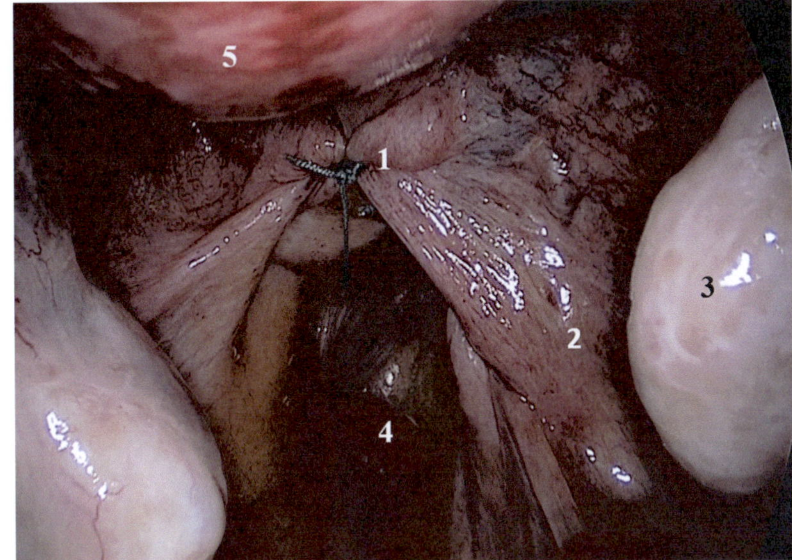

Fig. 6.25 Causes of ureteric injury. Surgery for pelvic organ prolapse. Descending course of the ureters (dashed red lines). Vaginal reconstructive surgery for a stage 4 pelvic organ prolapse. The blue area represents the reflection of the bladder through the anterior vaginal wall. (1) Bladder (after colpectomy), (2) exteriorized cervix, (3) anterior vaginal wall cut

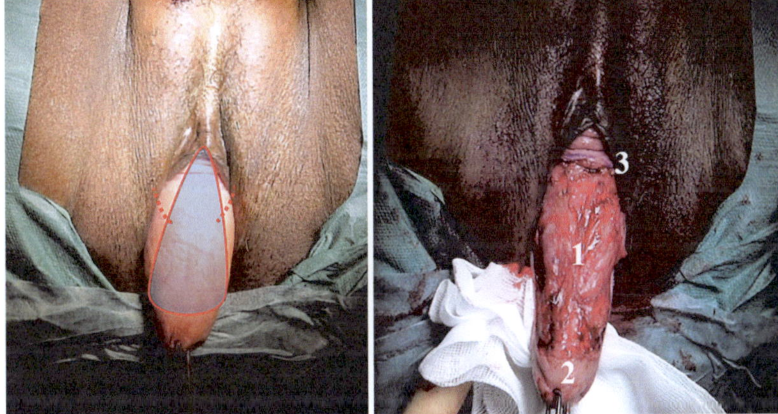

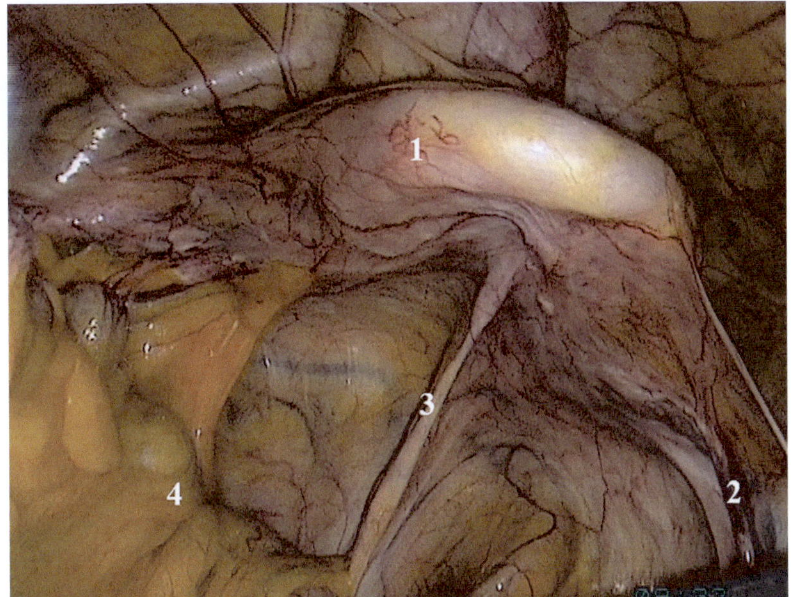

Fig. 6.26 Causes of ureteric injury: Pelvic organ prolapse treatment. Exteriorized vaginal vault prolapse. Laparoscopic view. (1) Vaginal vault pushed up using a vaginal retractor introduced transvaginally, (2) right ureter, (3) cul-de-sac of Douglas with large enterocele, (4) bowel

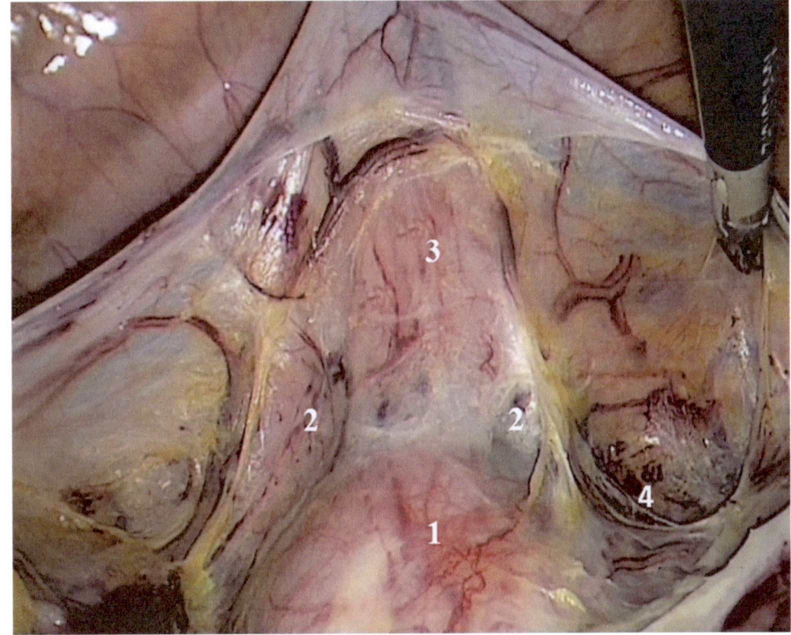

Fig. 6.27 Causes of ureteric injury. Surgery of pelvic organ prolapse. Deep laparoscopic vesicovaginal cleavage. The ureter is under the level of the bladder pillar and lateral (1) Vagina, (2) bladder pillar, (3) bladder (lifted), (4) area of the right ureter, lateral (not seen)

6.9 Stress Urinary Incontinence Treatment (Figs. 6.28 and 6.29)

During the Burch procedure, colpopexy is performed by access to the Retzius space. The risk of injury to the ureter is low because the suspension sutures are fixed at the level of the urethrovesical junction and far from the trigone (Fig. 6.28).

There is a possible risk of kinking the ureter during laparoscopic colpopexy. After dissection of the Retzius space, the sutures are placed from the fascia covering the vagina (close to the external limit of the bladder) to the Cooper ligament. The dorsal sutures may have too much tension, kinking the ureter (Fig. 6.29).

6.10 Obstetrical Practice

During cesarean section or postpartum hysterectomy for severe hemorrhage, the injury of the ureter is rare: 0.09% ureteral lesion for Eisenkop et al. [12], 0.027% for Rajasekar et al. [13].

During a cesarean section, the ureter is usually injured when the hysterotomy accidentally extends either to the broad ligament or below the bladder. The ureter can be damaged during blind hemostasis and uterine wall closure, the vision being impaired by blood and clots. The left ureter (more ventral) is the most exposed due to dextrorotation of the pregnant uterus.

In the long series of 5619 caesarean sections, Lo et al. [14] observed a ureteral lesion in 0.1% of cases, recognized postoperatively, including three re-interventions immediately afterward for acute abdomen with uretero-uterine fistula, and three remote treatment. The treatment was ureteroneocystostomy in one case, flap ureteroneocystostomy according to Boari in one case, transureteroureterostomy in one case, and maintenance of a prolonged ureteral catheter in one case. The injuries occurred five out of six times on the left ureter.

6.11 In Summary of Iatrogenic Lesions of the Ureter

Benign gynecological procedures and malignant surgical treatments where ureteral injury can occur are varied. However, there are risk factors during gynecological surgery [15].

The main risk factors associated with ureteral injury are:

- Intraoperative hemorrhage.
- Large uterus filling and obstructing the pelvis.
- Ovarian neoplasms.
- Previous pelvic surgeries have caused severe adhesions between the pelvic organs and made difficult access to the uterine pedicles or ovaries.
- Severe pelvic adhesions and distorted pelvic anatomy.
- Severe endometriosis including the ureter.
- Radical hysterectomy.
- High-grade anterior compartment prolapse with difficulty in locating the ureter.
- Ectopic insertion of the ureter in the bladder.
- History of pelvic irradiation.

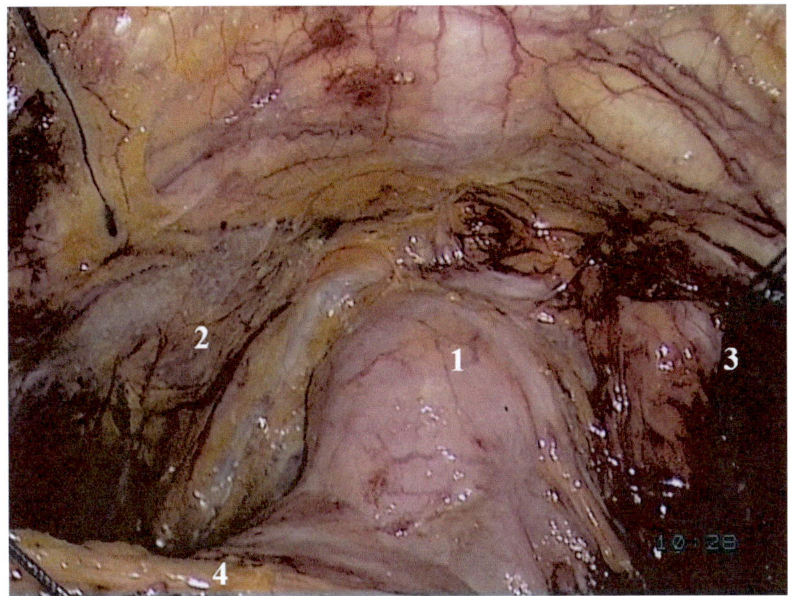

Fig. 6.28 Causes of ureteric injury: Stress urinary incontinence treatment: During incontinence treatment of Burch colposuspension procedure or of anterior compartment procedure. In this view, we see on the right side the suspension of the endopelvic fascia to the Cooper ligament with non-absorbable sutures. The passage of the sutures are lateral to the bladder and the ureter is posterior to the lateral dissection. On the left side, the suspension is not still done. (1) Bladder, (2) endopelvic fascia covering laterally the vagina, (3) Retzius space after dissection and colposuspension, (4) uterus

Fig. 6.29 Stress urinary incontinence: During performing Burch colposuspension or anterior compartment procedures, kinking the ureter is rare. (1) Burch procedure, (2) Cooper ligament, (3) bladder, (4) obturator muscle, (5) ureter is far after sufficient dissection

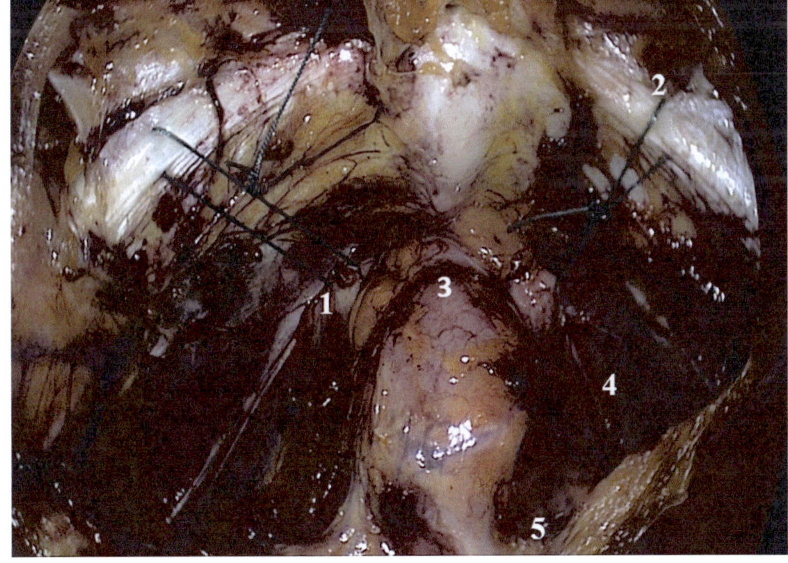

References

1. Solomons E, Levin EJ, Bauman J, Baron J. A Pyelographic study of ureteric injuries sustained during hysterectomy for benign conditions. Surg Gynecol Obstet. 1960;111:41–8.
2. Harkki-Siren P, Sjoberg J, Tiitinen A. Urinary tract injuries after hysterectomy. Obstet Gynecol. 1998;92(1):113–8.
3. Makinen J, Johansson J, Tomas C, Tomas E, Heinonen PK, Laatikainen T, Kauko M, Heikkinen AM, Sjoberg J. Morbidity of 10 110 hysterectomies by type of approach. Hum Reprod. 2001;16(7):1473–8.
4. Chapron C, Dubuisson JB, Ansquer Y, Fernandez B. Total hysterectomy for benign pathologies. Laparoscopic surgery does not seem to increase the risk of complications. J Gynecol Obstet Biol Reprod (Paris). 1998;27(1):55–61.
5. Adelman MR, Bardsley TR, Sharp HT. Urinary tract injuries in laparoscopic hysterectomy: a systematic review. J Minim Invasive Gynecol. 2014;21(4):558–66.
6. Gilmour DT, Das S, Flowerdew G. Rates of urinary tract injury from gynecologic surgery and the role of intraoperative cystoscopy. Obstet Gynecol. 2006;107:1366–72.
7. Kiran A, Hilton P, Cromwell DA. The risk of ureteric injury associated with hysterectomy, a 10-year retrospective cohort study. BJOG. 2016;123(7):1184–91.
8. Li F, Guo H, Qiu H, Liu S, Wang K, Yang C, Zheng TC, Q, Hou Y. Urologic complications after radical hysterectomy with postoperative radiotherapy and radiotherapy alone for cervical cancer. Medicine (Baltimore). 2018;97(13):e0173.
9. Hesselmann S, Hogberg U, Jonsson M. Effect of remote cesarean delivery on complications during hysterectomy: a cohort study. Am J Obstet Gynecol. 2017;217(5):564.e1–8.
10. Chang EJ, Mandelbaum RS, Nusbaum DJ, Violette CJ, Matsushima K, Klar M, Matsuzaki S, Machida H, Kanao H, Roman LD, Matsuo K. Vesivoureteral injury during benign hysterectomy: Minimally invasive laparoscopic surgery versus laparotomy. J Minim Invasive Gynecol. 2020;27(6):1354–62.
11. Alves J, Puga M, Fernandes R, Pinton A, Miranda I, Kovoor E, Wattiez A. Laparoscopic management of ureteral endometriosis and hydronephrosis associated with endometriosis. J Minim Invasive Gynecol. 2017;24(3):466–72.
12. Eisenkop SM, Richman R, Platt LD, Paul RH. Urinary tract injury during cesarean section. Obstet Gynecol. 1982;60(5):591–6.
13. Rajasekar D, Hall M. Urinary tract injuries during the obstetric intervention. Br J Obstet Gynaecol. 1997;104(6):731–4.
14. Lo TS, Wijaya T, Kao CC, Wu PY, Cortes EFM, Huang SY, Lin CH. Clinical relevance and treatment selection of ureteral injury after cesarean section. Female Pelvic Med Reconstr Surg. 2016;22(5):303–6.
15. Dandolu V, Mathai E, Chatwani A, Harmanli O, Pontari M, Hernandez E. Accuracy of cystoscopy in the diagnosis of ureteral injury in benign gynecologic surgery. Int Urogynecol J Pelvic Floor Dysfunct. 2003;14(6):427–31.

## Part III

Prevention, Diagnosis, and Treatment of Traumatic Lesions of the Ureter

Prevention of Traumatic Lesions of the Ureter During Gynecological Surgery

7

J.-B. Dubuisson et al., *Ureteral Complications of Gynecological Surgery*,
https://doi.org/10.1007/978-3-031-15598-7_7

Chapter 7 concerns the prevention of the traumatic lesions of the ureter during pelvic surgery. It is one of the more fundamental aspects of this book. The first part includes the usual recommendations in gynecological surgery according to the principles of the ureter anatomy and the most frequent pathologies and surgical procedures.

The second part concerns special recommendations for laparoscopic hysterectomy, including fenestration of the broad ligament, uterine manipulator use, hemostasis of the uterine vessels, and bladder cleavage. Finally, other recommendations are discussed in the most difficult conditions.

7.1　Usual Recommendations

The first step of any gynecological operation is a precise preoperative assessment of the pathology. If it seems difficult, we should consider abdominal ultrasound, MRI, CT scan with contrast, rarely intravenous urogram (IVU). After that, an appropriate operative approach may be performed.

These recommendations are only of interest for gynecological operations where one of the intraoperative procedures is performed near the ureter.

The main rule is to always visualize both ureters. If this is not possible, the ureters should be palpated with the finger (or rather between two fingers) during a laparotomy or vaginal surgery. It is spotted using atraumatic forceps during a laparoscopy. Gentle pressure on the ureter is enough to see it crawling (Kelly's sign). In case of visualization failure, ureterolysis is recommended [1].

Visualization of the ureter is easy by longitudinal incision of the parietal peritoneum lateral to the infundibulopelvic ligament, giving access to retroperitoneal structures.

It is important to avoid separating the ureter from the peritoneum which is adherent to it. Leaving as much of the ureter as possible adherent to the normally attached peritoneum is needed.

General rules for ureterolysis are well defined. The longitudinally running blood vessels should be preserved by the inclusion of a few millimeters of tissue around the ureter (mesoureter). So, T-shaped arteries and vertically running branches should not be interrupted.

The use of electrocoagulation and diathermy should be moderate, just as necessary. Near the ureter, we should do only short applications of low voltage diathermy. We have also to take care of the manipulation of the ureter after the use of hot bipolar forceps, ultrasound, or vessel-sealing device. Cooling the hot instruments before touching the ureter area is recommended.

7.1.1　Ureter and Pelvic Tumor

Large pelvic tumors, even though nonmalignant, modify pelvic anatomy and the ureter may be displaced or compressed. Large leiomyomas and ovarian cysts may be associated with hydroureter and hydronephrosis. These tumors displace the ureter down and laterally or down and medially.

In the case of a pelvic tumor, it is recommended to identify the ureter at the level of the promontory, in healthy tissue, so at distance, and then follow it to the tumor. In theory, it's easy, but in practice, it is more difficult, especially in case of hemorrhagic dissection or severe adhesions.

7.1.2　Dissection Plane

During dissection of the ureter, it is preferable to leave tissue around it (adventitia and mesoureter) to protect the T-shaped arteries and thus avoid any devascularization.

7.1.3 Bladder Pillars

During an open hysterectomy, the mobilization of the bladder separates the lower uterine segment from the bladder; the bladder pillars are an upper landmark. It is recommended to avoid descending lower, especially in total hysterectomy for a benign pathology. The issue is different in the case of radical hysterectomy or oncologic surgery where tumor resection may be deeper, with dissection of the vesicouterine ligament and ureteric tunnel.

7.1.4 Hemostasis of Uterine Vessels

During a standard hysterectomy, hemostasis is a performed flush with the cervix. Dextrorotation of the uterus may explain why the left ureter is more at risk of injury than the right.

7.1.5 Intraligamentous Uterine Leiomyoma

In intraligamentous uterine leiomyoma, the ureter is usually located below and outward.

The incision of the peritoneum is made just above the pedicle or on the dome of the leiomyoma and allows the intracapsular enucleation to be carried out safely, away from the ureter. The risk of ureteral injury occurs especially during accidental hemorrhage including difficult and blind hemostasis. It is the reason why the preventive occlusion of the ipsilateral uterine artery, 4 cm dorsally to the crossing of the ureter or close to its origin is recommended, limiting the bleeding during the dissection of the leiomyoma. The peritoneal incision lateral to the infundibulopelvic ligament gives access to the external iliac artery and more medially to the ureter.

7.1.6 Ureter and Ovarian Cyst

In the case of an ovarian cyst, the ureter is below and medially. But if the cyst grows below the lower edge of the ovarian fossa, the ureter may be raised and be on the upper surface of the cyst, making it more vulnerable. Observation and palpation are always necessary before dissection, even in the case of a benign ovarian cyst.

7.2 Special Recommendations for Laparoscopic Hysterectomy

7.2.1 Surgeon Experience

Wattiez et al. [2] stressed the importance of the surgeon's experience regarding risk limitation during laparoscopic hysterectomy. Thus, in this study comparing two successive series, only two cases out of 952 were observed in the second series 1996–1999 during which the surgical team had experience, against 4 out of 695 in the first series 1989–1995. It means the importance of training to observe a low rate of complications.

7.2.2 Fenestration of the Broad Ligament (Figs. 7.1 and 7.2)

After traction of the round ligament and its coagulation section, fenestration of the broad ligament by an incision in the pars flaccida, just below the tube and the ovarian ligament, releases the ureter downward with the peritoneum (Fig. 7.1).

This technique makes it possible to coagulate and cut safely the infundibulopelvic ligament with ovarian vessels away from the ureter. It makes it easy to cut and coagulate the Fallopian tube and utero-ovarian ligament (Fig. 7.2).

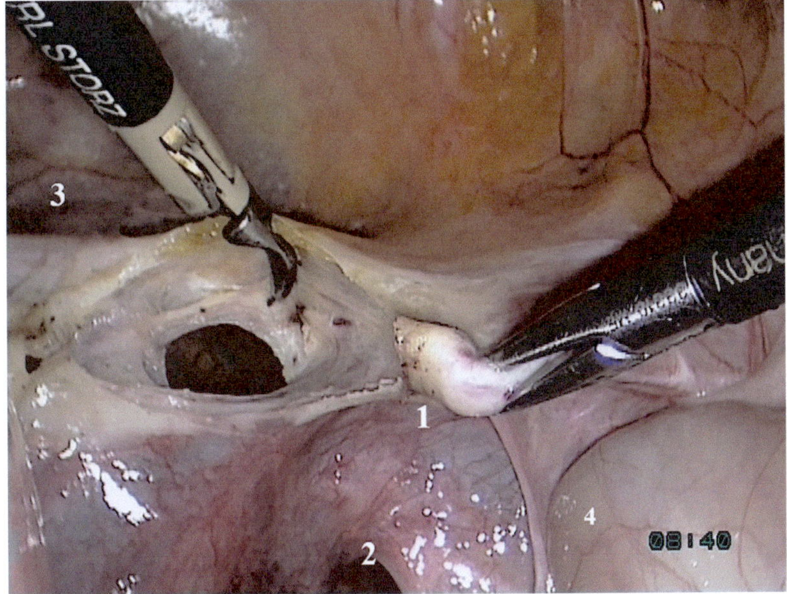

Fig. 7.1 Prevention of ureteric injury during laparoscopic hysterectomy. Initial fenestration of the broad ligament. Right side. (1) Round ligament transsected, (2) tube, (3) bladder, (4) bowel

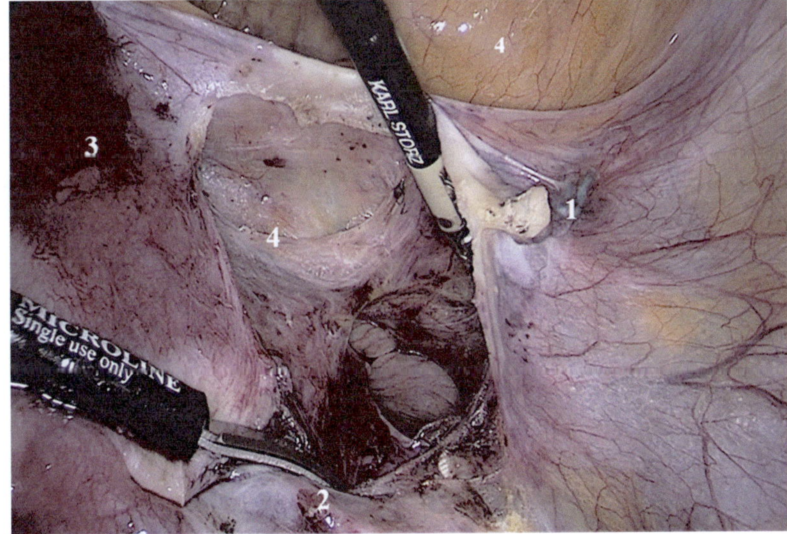

Fig. 7.2 Prevention of ureteric injury during laparoscopic hysterectomy. Initial fenestration of the broad ligament. Right side. (1) round ligament, (2) tube, (3) uterus, (4) bladder

7.2.3 Comfort Obtained with the Uterine Manipulator (Fig. 7.3)

The use of a uterine manipulator combining an intrauterine cannula and an intravaginal cup makes it possible to safely mobilize and push the uterus upward. This moves up the uterine pedicles and frees them from the bladder and ureters for dissection. Regarding the height of the occlusion of the uterine artery, it is always done at the level of the internal opening of the cervix, or visually at the level of the torus uterinum. It is 1.5 cm medial to the ureter. Ligation of the descending branches of the uterine artery is done flush with the cervix. The vaginal cup of the manipulator allows circular colpotomy in better safety using a monopolar hook, a monopolar needle, or scissors.

7.2.4 Ureter and Hemostasis of the Uterine Vessels (Fig. 7.4)

By laparoscopy, the coagulation of the uterine vessels is usually done using bipolar forceps or a vessel sealer device. The placement of the forceps should be done away from the ureter to prevent any hazardous thermal diffusion. All types of electrosurgical instruments can cause substantial thermal injury to surrounding tissues by thermal spread. It includes monopolar hooks or scissors, bipolar forceps, harmonic scalpels, and vessel sealer devices. For the latter, thermal energy diffuses up to 3 mm; up to 10 mm for standard bipolar forceps, depending on the power settings and the duration of application. If you use this type of energy, you must know its theoretical principles and be as careful as with other techniques [3]. So, it should be important to stay close to the cervix for hemostasis of the uterine vessels. Dextrorotation of the uterus may explain that the left ureter is more often damaged than the right.

By laparoscopy or laparotomy, blind hemostatic clamping or blind coagulation neither should be performed. In case of an injured uterine artery or of its branches with active bleeding, it is important to identify quickly the site of bleeding. Compression with a swab is done or with digital compression (laparotomy) or pressure with a laparoscopic atraumatic forceps (laparoscopy). Then, after aspiration of the blood, coagulation or ligation of the uterine artery is done above the bleeding vessel. Finally, without active bleeding, hemostasis can be safely achieved.

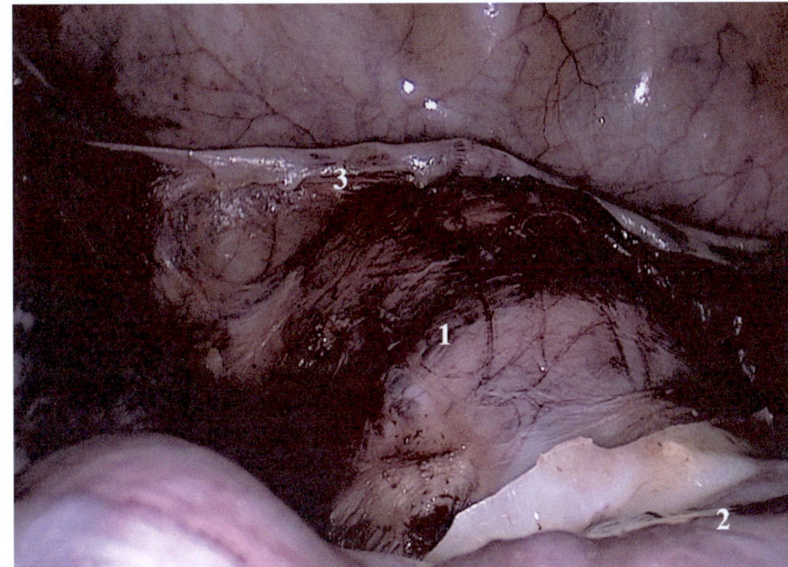

Fig. 7.3 Prevention of ureteric injury during laparoscopic total hysterectomy. The use of a uterine manipulator to push the uterus upward. (1) Vaginal cup of the uterine manipulator well visible below the anterior wall of the vagina, (2) uterus, (3) bladder

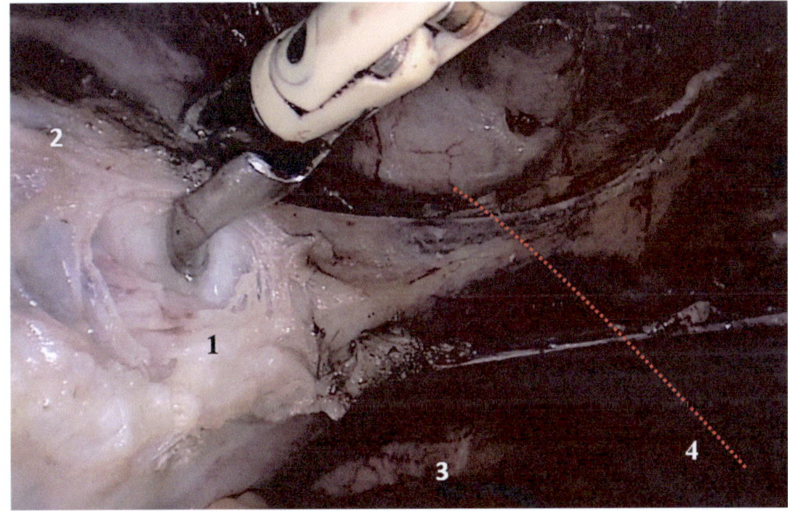

Fig. 7.4 Prevention of ureteric injury during laparoscopic hysterectomy. Hemostasis of the uterine vessels. Artery coagulation at a precise level. Right side. Presumed ureteral course (dashed red lines). (1) Coagulation of the uterine pedicle, (2) uterus, (3) uterosacral ligament, (4) ureter

7.2.5 Precise Level for the Treatment of the Uterine Pedicle (Fig. 7.5)

The coagulation of the uterine pedicle is performed at the precise level: back at the level of the torus uterinum, forward above the bladder pillars.

7.2.6 Ureter and Bladder (Fig. 7.6)

It is important to have sufficient safety for the ureter during bladder mobilization. It is necessary to control, separate, and repress the bladder sufficiently before the colpotomy. The vaginal cup of the uterine manipulator helps to find the correct plane. In case of a difficult vesicovaginal cleavage with the poor vision of the caudal edge of the bladder, the surgeon may fill the bladder with serum and indigo carmine with the bladder catheter. The view of a "blue and filled bladder" makes easier the dissection between bladder and vagina.

Fig. 7.5 Prevention of ureteric injury during laparoscopic hysterectomy. Precise level of coagulation-section of the uterine pedicles. Right side. Presumed ureteral course (dashed red lines), uterine manipulator in place. (1) Devascularized uterus, (2) uterine vessels transsected, (3) uterosacral ligament, (4) vaginal cup pushing the uterus upwards (torus uterinum), (5) bladder, (6) presumed ureteral course

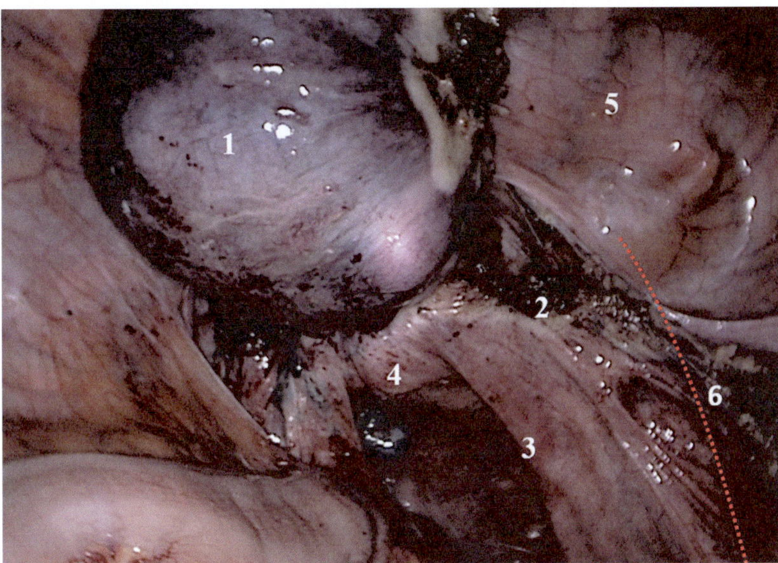

Fig. 7.6 Prevention of ureteric injury during laparoscopic hysterectomy. Bladder dissection. (1) Bladder, (2) limit of the bladder, (3) vagina with the relief of the cup, (4) uterus

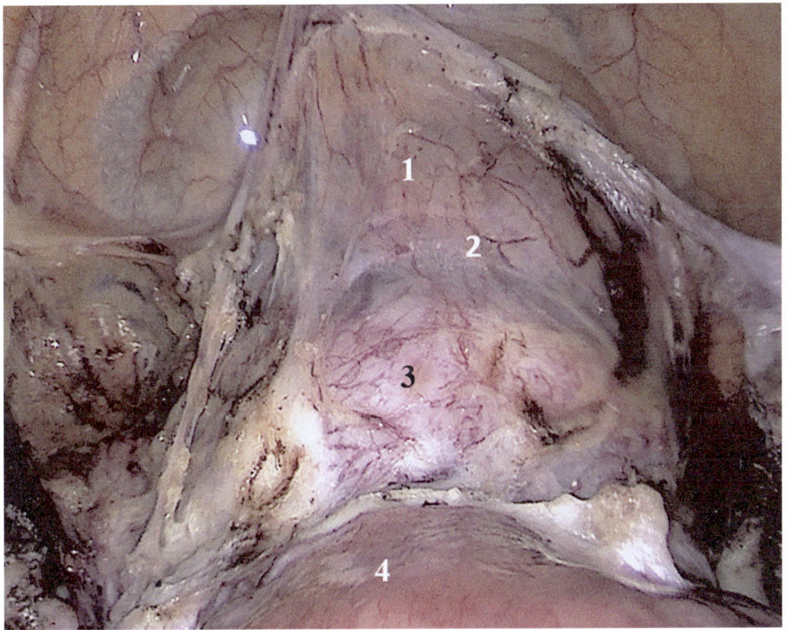

7.2.7 Limited Dissection of the Broad Ligament (Fig. 7.7)

During hysterectomy for benign pathology, there is a limited dissection of the broad ligament with separation of the anterior and the posterior leaves at a distance from the ureter.

7.2.8 Closure of the Peritoneum

Often, in the difficult cases of radical pelvic surgery and even hysterectomy, the peritoneum cannot be closed correctly. The operated area should be left open, avoiding any kinking of the ureter.

7.3 Prevention of Ureteral Injury During Surgery for Endometriosis (Fig. 7.8)

The ureter is visualized before any excision or coagulation of the endometriotic implant or nodule.

Sometimes the ureter may be visible and followed under the peritoneum, by transparency.

If the adhesions are severe and extensive, the visualization of the ureter is not possible. The opening of the peritoneum and its horizontal incision just medial to the infundibulopelvic ligament (endometriosis approach) offers a direct gentle dissection of the ureter. Then, ureterolysis may be performed.

Fig. 7.7 Prevention of ureteric injury during laparoscopic hysterectomy. The limited dissection of the broad ligament. Anterior and posterior leaves are separated. Right side. (1) Uterus, (2) tube (transsected), (3) broad ligament, (4) uterosacral ligament, (5) round ligament (transsected)

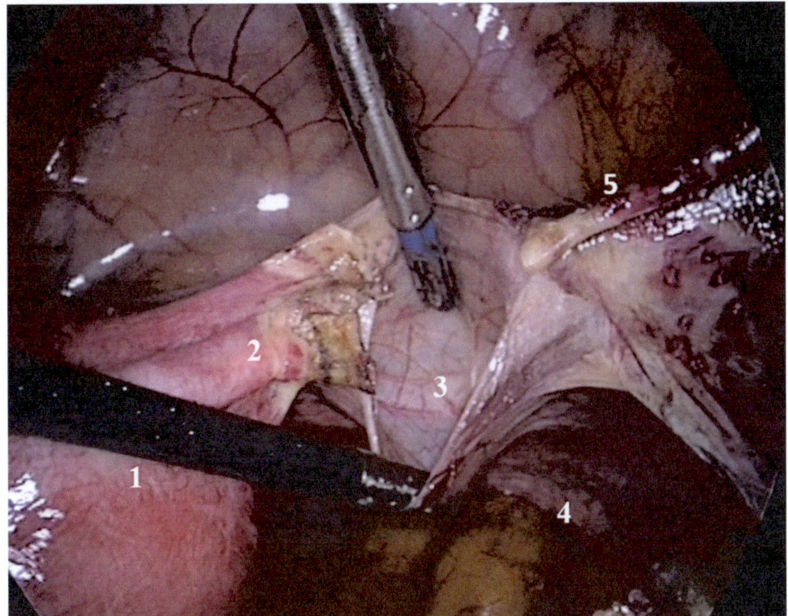

Fig. 7.8 Prevention of ureteric injury during laparoscopic surgery for endometriosis. Visualization of the ureter. Right side. (1) Ureter, (2) uterosacral ligament with endometriotic lesions, (3) bowel

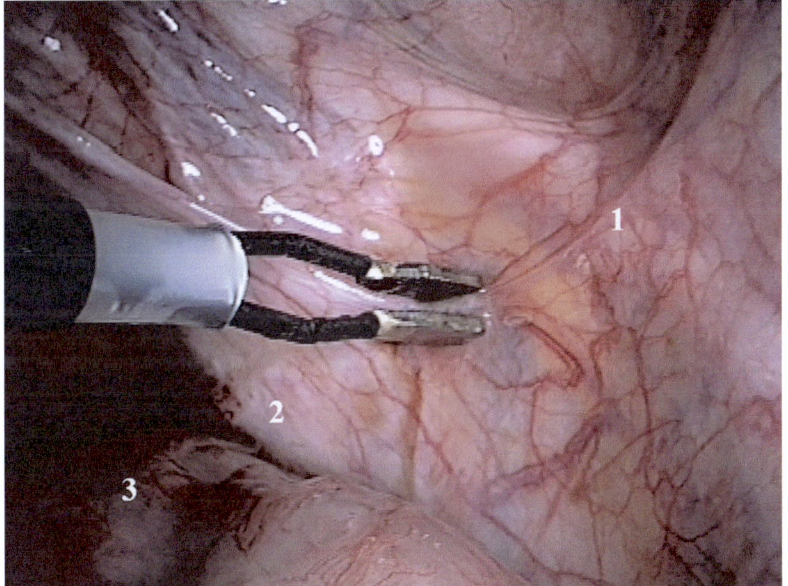

7.4   Prevention of Ureteral Injury During Occlusion of the Uterine Artery
(Figs. 7.9 and 7.10)

Occlusion of the uterine artery at its origin (4 cm dorsally to the crossing) may be a security to prevent bleeding during complex hysterectomy, especially with huge volume, and myomectomy of large leiomyomas (Fig. 7.9). At this level, it is quite easy to dissect the uterine artery from the ureter.

The occlusion of the uterine artery with a Titanium clip (or a Bulldog clamp) is easy and better than using coagulation with forceps because of the risk of thermal diffusion and consequently potential burn of the ureter (Fig. 7.10).

Fig. 7.9 Prevention of ureteric injury during laparoscopic occlusion of the uterine artery. Right side. (1) Ureter, (2) uterine artery (site of occlusion), (3) uterosacral ligament

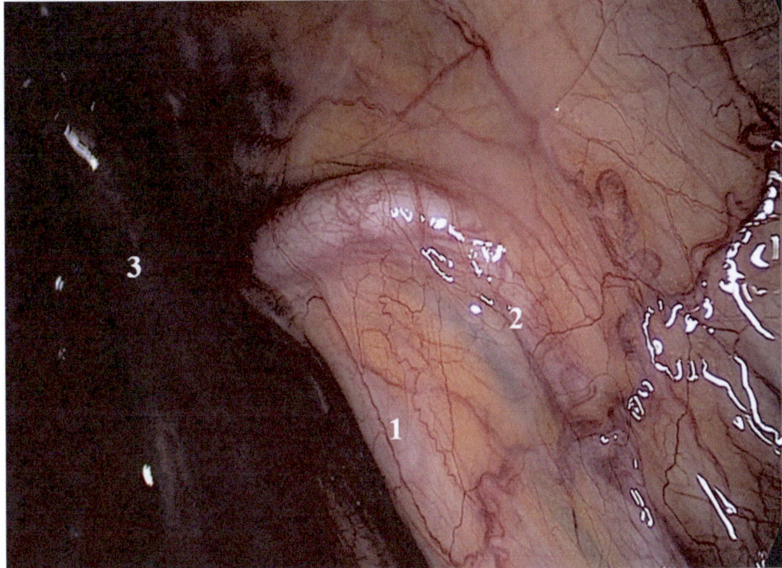

Fig. 7.10 Prevention of ureteric injury. During upper occlusion of the uterine artery with a titanium clip. Right side. Occlusion of the uterine artery using a titanium clip. (1) Ureter, (2) uterine artery with clip (white arrow), (3) tube

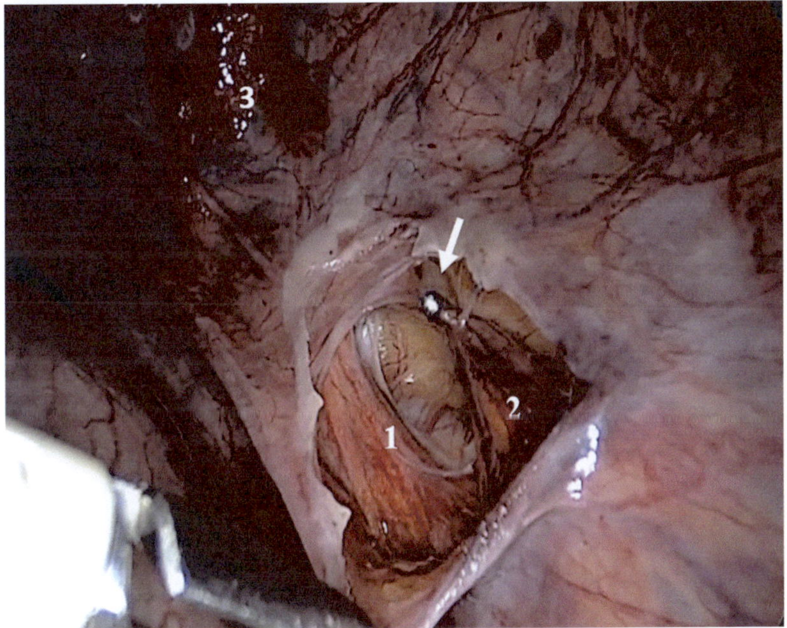

7.5 Prevention of Ureteral Injury in the Presence of Anatomical Anomalies (Fig. 7.11)

The surgeon must be aware of anatomical anomalies of the pelvis during the initial inspection. For instance, precise observation can demonstrate the absence of a uterosacral ligament. The ureter may be mistaken for a uterosacral ligament that is absent.

7.6 Prevention of Ureteral Injury During High Plications of the Uterosacral Ligaments or McCall Procedure for Pelvic Reconstruction (Fig. 7.12)

The passage of the curved needle into the uterosacral ligaments and nearby tissues should be away from the ureter, which course must be identified at the level of the suture. In case of doubt about kinking the ureter, limited ureterolysis to push away the ureter must be performed.

7.7 Prevention During Cesarean Section and Postpartum Hysterectomy for Hemorrhage

The risk of ureter injury during cesarean section is rare. During a hysterectomy performed for important bleeding, the blood interferes with vision in the operative field. The situation of the ureter during pregnancy and delivery with the enlargement of the cervix increases the risk. It is more evident for the left ureter because of the dextrorotation of the uterus. It is more anterior than the right ureter and more vulnerable. Exteriorization of the uterus out of the pelvis could help to recognize anatomical structures and limit the risk of ureteric injury. Palpation of the ureter or ureterolysis could help in case of bleeding in the lateral parametrium area.

Presumed course of the left ureter (red dashed line). (1) Culdoplasty, (2) left ureter, (3) left uterosacral ligament, (4) rectum

Fig. 7.11 Prevention of ureteric injury. Beware of anatomical anomalies. (1) Right uterosacral ligament, (2) absence of left uterosacral ligament, (3) cul-de-sac of Douglas, (4) torus uterinum, (5) uterus, (6) left ureter

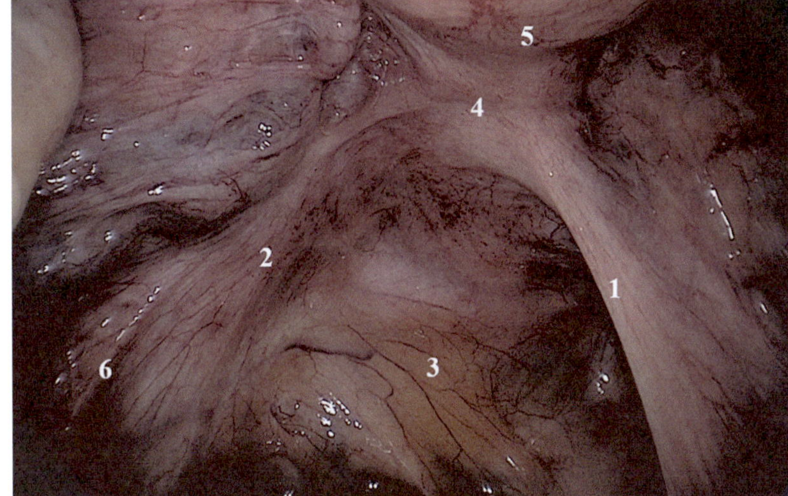

Fig. 7.12 Prevention of ureteric injuries during laparoscopic high plications of uterosacral ligament and culdoplasty according to McCall procedure for pelvic reconstruction

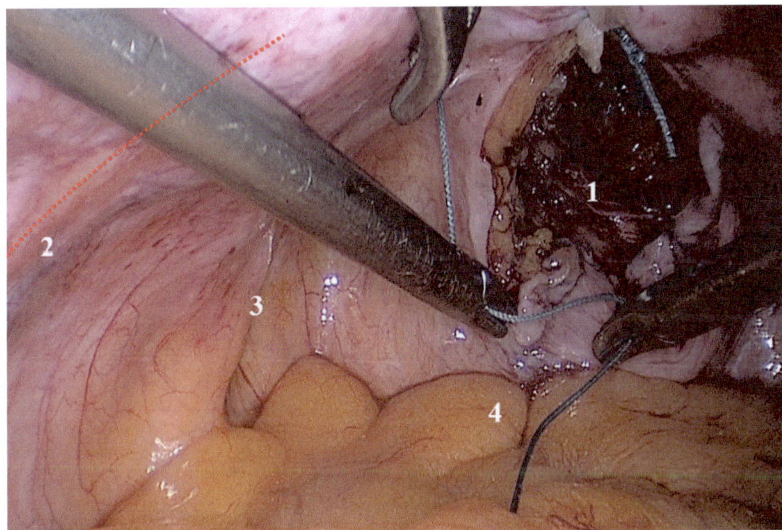

References

1. Jan H, Ghai V. Ureterolysis for Laparoscopic Hysterectomy. J Minim Invasive Gynecol. 2019;26(3):401.
2. Wattiez A, Soriano D, Cohen SB, Nervo P, Canis M, Botchorishvili R, et al. The learning curve of total laparoscopic hysterectomy: comparative analysis of 1647 cases. J Am Assoc Gynecol Laparosc. 2002;9(3):339–45.
3. Liang J, Xing H, Chang Y. Thermal damage width and hemostatic effect of bipolar electrocoagulation, LigaSure, and Ultracision techniques on goat mesenteric vessels and optimal power for bipolar electrocoagulation. BMC Surg. 2019;19(1):147.

What to Do during the Operation in the Event of a Suspected Ureteral Lesion?

Chapter 8 concerns the management of a suspected iatrogenic lesion during a gynecological operation. It is one of the major and stressful issues for the surgeon. The additional surgical procedures needed to help him to have a precise diagnosis are discussed, i.e., intravenous injection of indigo carmine, cystoscopy, visualization of the course of the ureter, and precise recognition of the iatrogenic lesion.

The ureteral lesion can be suspected in case of visualization of a dilated ureter and/or reduced ureteral peristalsis. In rare cases including the ureteral section, propulsion of urine into the abdominal cavity out of a "tube" can be seen.

First, it is important to follow the course of the ureter all the way and inspect it. Ureterolysis can then be performed, starting in healthy tissue.

Second, the surgeon should strongly consider contacting the urologist.

8.1   Intravenous Injection of Indigo Carmine at the Slightest Suspicion

Initially developed as a textile dye in the mid-eighteenth century, indigo carmine has been used as a food colorant and pH indicator. After intravenous administration of a standard dose (5 ml of 0.4%, i.e., 20 mg) it is rapidly cleared by the kidneys without further metabolization, giving urine an intense blue color after approximately 10 min. For added efficacy, it can be associated with intravenous furosemide administration.

The injection of indigo carmine can help detect a ureteral fistula, in case of open access or laparoscopy, if there is any doubt about damage to the ureter. During laparotomy or laparoscopy, in the event of a fistula or ureteral section, a blue liquid flow will therefore be seen in the abdominal cavity. There are no common contraindications to its use apart from previous adverse reactions.

8.2   During Cystoscopy (Figs. 8.1, 8.2 and 8.3)

Cystoscopy visualizes all the bladder cavities (Fig. 8.1). Bladder integrity is checked and then the two ureteric orifices.

The ejaculation of urine through ureteric orifices is well seen (Fig. 8.2).

A large opening of the ureteric orifice can be observed during ejaculation (Fig. 8.3). Following the injection of indigo carmine, the "blue" color is observed during the first 10 min. Furosemide potentiates the test by increasing urine output. Normally, the cystoscopy at the end of the operation shows the passage of indigo carmine through the two ostia symmetrically. It is useful at the end of a complex hysterectomy or after a Burch procedure or ureterolysis. For some surgeons, cystoscopy with indigo carmine is performed systematically at the end of a laparoscopic hysterectomy.

Cystoscopy with indigo carmine appears to have good sensitivity for the detection of ureteral obstruction and bladder lesions. Gilmour DT et al. [1] reviewed 47 studies on complications of the urinary tract after surgery. The incidence varies from 1 per 1000 without cystoscopy and 13 per 1000 in case of systematic cystoscopy. Gilmour et al. [1] also report that in the 18 series using systematically cystoscopy with indigo carmine after gynecological surgery, the rate of intraoperative detection of ureteral and bladder lesions were 89% and 95%, respectively.

However, it can give false information in cases of incomplete stenosis. In these cases of incomplete stenosis, the cystoscopy often shows asymmetry of the flow of indigo carmine in the bladder, at the level of the ureteral orifices, which will require further investigation.

Fig. 8.1 What to do in case of intraoperative doubt about a ureteric injury. Cystoscopy. Exploration of the entire bladder and locating the orifices. *: Left ureteric orifice

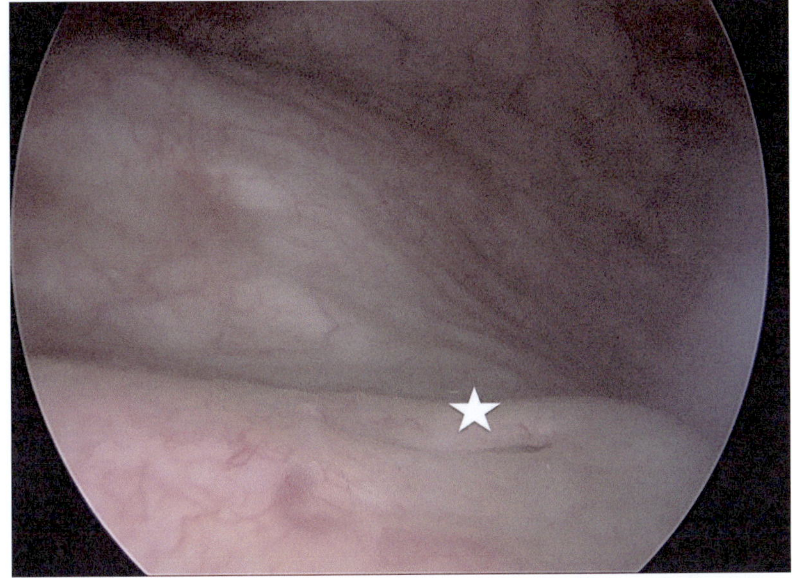

Fig. 8.2 What to do in case of intraoperative doubt about a ureteric injury. Cystoscopy. Passage of urine in the bladder (white arrow)

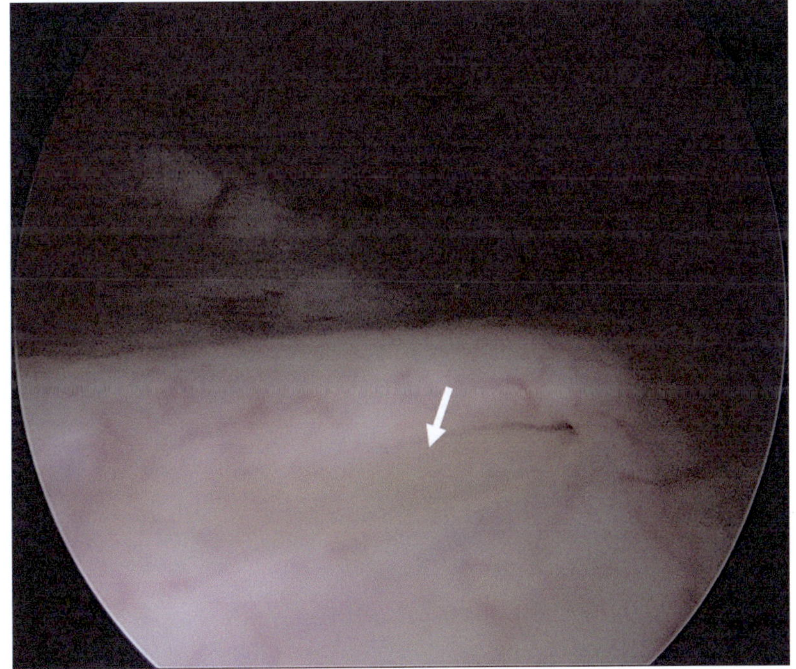

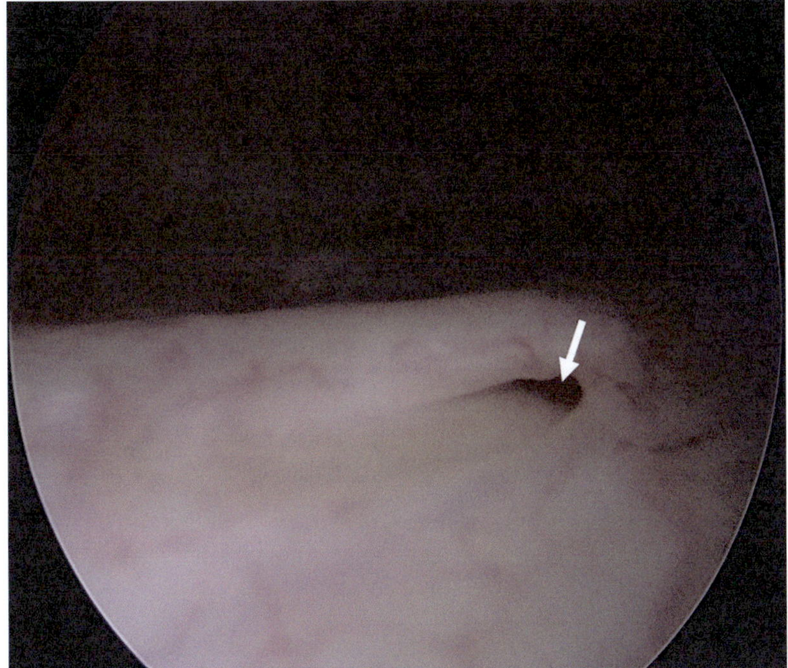

Fig. 8.3 What to do in case of intraoperative doubt about a ureteric injury. Cystoscopy. Large opening of the ureteric orifice (white arrow)

8.3 Recognition of an Intraoperative Complication

8.3.1 Thread Ligation

If there is significant doubt about the stenosis made by thread ligation, ureterolysis should be done first. Dissection of the ureter is followed by a section of the thread responsible for the stenosis and then evaluation of the ureter. If the ureter is unharmed, abstention is required. If the compression is visible or the wall of the ureter is damaged, the immediate fitting of the JJ ureteral stent is recommended.

8.3.2 Thermal Injury

If in doubt about a burn, the ureter is first released. The burn is rarely authenticated by discoloration or perforation of the ureter. It is treated, if possible, by immediately rise of a ureteral stent.

8.3.3 Section of the Ureter

In the event of a blunt section, precise local hemostasis must be ensured, avoiding devascularization of the ureter, and then performing either a ureteroureterostomy (end-to-end anastomosis) or an immediate ureteroneocystostomy (reimplantation).

Partial transection of the ureter is repaired by a few sutures over a ureteric stent.

Reference

1. Gilmour DT, Das S, Flowerdew G. Rates of urinary tract injury from gynecologic surgery and the role of intraoperative cystoscopy. Obstet Gynecol. 2006;107:1366–72.

What to Do after Surgery in Case of the Suspected Ureteral Lesion?

J.-B. Dubuisson et al., *Ureteral Complications of Gynecological Surgery*,
https://doi.org/10.1007/978-3-031-15598-7_9

Chapter 9 concerns the postoperative course of a gynecological operation when an iatrogenic ureter lesion is suspected. The place of imaging is very important. The complication is sometimes difficult to diagnose.

This chapter is a long discussion including the clinical signs suggesting a postoperative complication, i.e., obstruction or fistula, and the different aspects of imaging.

The principles of treatment are to restore patency and ureter tightness and to drain the retroperitoneal space in the event of a urinoma.

9.1 Clinical Signs Suggesting a Postoperative Complication

These can range from fully asymptomatic situations to a frank uroperitoneum with uremia and shock.

9.1.1 Ureter Obstruction

In the case of ureteral obstruction, symptoms may be absent or mild in incomplete cases. A diagnosis will then be made incidentally on imaging or due to elevated serum creatinine or BUN (blood urea nitrogen). These can still be within the normal range but noticeably increased compared to preoperative values. In more severe cases, one may expect continuous and dull flank pain linked with renal distension. Depending on the height of the obstruction, it may be present in the lower lateral quadrant and extend into the groin. Rarely, the clinical presentation can mimic acute renal colic and cause a pyelic rupture at most. Generally, symptoms will be less obvious due to postoperative analgesia or be mistaken for normal postoperative pain. As always, a patient in pain should be carefully assessed.

9.1.2 Ureteral Leakage

In the case of urinary leakage, several scenarios are possible. A major intraperitoneal leak will cause urinary ascites. An ill-looking patient with diffuse abdominal discomfort and distension, ileus, oliguria, and profound azotemia will quickly undergo imaging. In case of lesser leaks, or leaks contained by adjacent structures or the retroperitoneum, the pain will be more localized and systemic signs more discrete. Persistent pain, low-grade fever, and abnormal elevated inflammatory or renal markers should lead to imaging. Typically, a urinary leak will be associated with some degree of ureteral obstruction and hydronephrosis. In case of major leaks without obstruction, imaging should reveal pelvic fluid collections or free intra-abdominal fluid.

If a drain is present, its output may stay persistently high. In case of doubt, creatinine or urea levels can be measured in its fluid. As these values can exceed usual serum levels over a thousand-fold, one should pay attention to the units used by the laboratory (they can seem normal at a first glance). After major pelvic surgery with abundant fluid accumulation and/or lymphorrhea, however, urinary metabolites may not be elevated even in the presence of leakage.

9.1.3 Ureter Fistula

Leakage of urine in the postoperative course is often mistaken for postoperative stress incontinence. It can be the indicator of a serious complication that needs to be managed quickly. After ruling out stress incontinence, a bladder or ureteral lesion should be suspected. The ureteral fistula accounts for approximately one-third of ureteral lesions following gynecologic surgery. Fistulation can be immediate or occur within 1 week. Urine is evacuated through the vagina (uterovaginal fistula after hysterectomy), through the uterus (uretero-uterine fistula after cesarean section), and drainage devices (drain aspiration, etc.). In ischemic ureteric involvement, fistulation is delayed, typically 2–3 weeks after surgery.

Generally, gross hematuria cannot be considered a reliable marker. Its consistent presence should lead to further investigations.

9.2 Imaging

9.2.1 Abdominal Ultrasound

In most situations, abdominal ultrasound will be the most readily available screening imaging in case of a suspected urinary tract complication.

Distension of the renal calyces, proximal and pelvis ureter will indicate a downstream obstruction, with or without additional leakage.

Free abdominal fluid or fluid collections in the pelvis can be reliably detected, without renal calyces distension in case of a complete ureteral or pyelic rupture.

The bladder or a correctly positioned urinary balloon catheter will be easily visible.

If present, the proximal and distal ends of ureteral stents should also be noticeable.

9.2.2 Ureteric Jet on Ultrasound

If the bladder is full enough, the ureteric jet, i.e., the flow of urine from the distal ureter into the bladder, can be recognized in grey-scale or color Doppler mode. In a well-hydrated, stable patient, it should occur at least twice per minute. Jet velocity can be measured, and low values have been associated with urine outflow obstruction. If in doubt, cross-sectional imaging should be performed.

9.2.3 Intravenous Urography

Rarely used nowadays, it consists of sequential abdominal plain film X-rays over 20 min after intravenous contrast administration. It allows the visualization of the renal parenchyma, collecting system, calyces, ureters, and bladder. An abdominal compression band is typically used to dilate and visualize the upper urinary tract in greater detail but should not be employed when a ureteral leak or obstruction is suspected.

9.2.4 CT Urography. Plain Film Abdominal X-Ray Following a Contrast-Enhanced CT Scan

CT urography evaluates kidneys, ureters, and bladder. It uses X-rays with multiple images of the different areas and finally, a 2D reconstruction is made. Performing a plain film of the abdomen in a supine position following CT urography will give an overview of the urinary system and help identify and locate anomalies in the urinary system. This can be of help if delayed, post-contrast phases were not acquired during the initial CT scan. In case of obstruction or leakage, contrast accumulation can be found even hours after the contrast administration.

This exam will visualize ureteral anomalies in the craniocaudal plane, i.e., the height of a ureteral lesion, which is of interest in the case of subsequent reconstructive surgery of the urinary tract.

9.2.5 MR Urography

MR urography provides a noninvasive visualization of the entire urinary tract, precisely the ureteral lesions and the integrity of the kidneys. It is quickly proposed in an emergency if the imagery center is well equipped with MRI machines.

9.2.6 ^{9m}Tc MAG3 Renal Scintigraphy

When imaging of the upper urinary tract can neither assert nor rule out the presence of significant ureteral obstruction, an MAG3 renal scan will be of help.

This dynamic imaging of the kidneys is based on technetium-labeled mercaptoacetyltriglycine, which is secreted by the renal tubules, followed by a timed diuretic injection. This study generates individual curves representing the three phases of the radionuclide's passage through each kidney: its renal uptake from the blood, parenchymal transit into the renal tubules, and its excretion into the collecting system with subsequent clearance into the ureters. In the case of ureteral obstruction, the renogram will keep rising or stagnating during the excretory phase. The degree of obstruction is then further assessed and quantified by the response to the diuretic. Furthermore, it weighs the relative renal function of each kidney, which can decrease in case of long-standing urinary obstruction.

The MAG3 renal scan is therefore a sensitive study to quantify the degree of urinary obstruction, in the presence of a mild renal dilation of unclear significance or as a follow-up study following ureteral reconstruction. It is however not a first-line diagnostic tool in case of acute ureteral injury.

9.2.7   Retrograde Pyelogram

As an endoscopic, fluoroscopic exam, a retrograde ureteropyelogram (short, retrograde pyelogram) can both be performed on shorthand notice during abdominal surgery or as a planned procedure. During the procedure, the distal ureter is catheterized under direct vision through a flexible or rigid cystoscope. Contrast liquid is then injected up the ureter into the renal pelvis and calyces.

It can be done in different types of patient positions using a flexible cystoscope, provided on the operating table which is radio translucent. If needed, a ureteral stent can be placed using the same access.

In an intact upper urinary tract, a retrograde pyelogram will reveal:

- the full length of the ureter, renal pelvis, and calyces,
- ureteral peristalsis,
- antegrade contrast secretion.

In abnormal situations, it can show:

- ureteral stenosis, leaks, or filling defects,
- adjacent radio-opaque structures such as staples,
- residual contrast agent from previous contrast-enhanced studies.

9.2.8   Iconography of Radiological Images (Figs. 9.1, 9.2, 9.3, 9.4, 9.5, 9.6, 9.7, 9.8, 9.9, 9.10, 9.11, 9.12 and 9.13)

Fig. 9.1 Intravenous urography. Absence of visualization of the left ureter (white arrow)

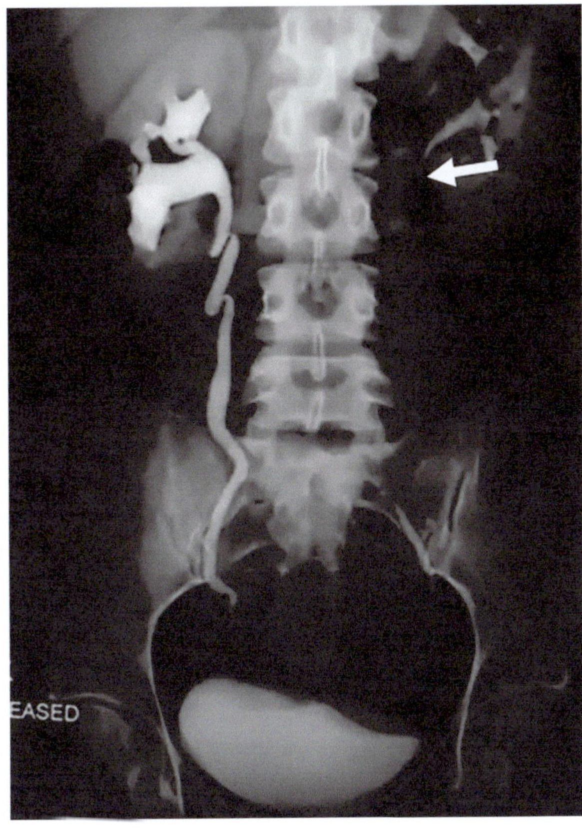

Fig. 9.2 Distal right ureteral kink. Partial obstruction during abdominal hysterectomy by laparotomy. First postoperative day. Kink by thread ligature. CT-scan: coronal reconstruction with excretion delay in the right kidney and stagnation of contrast medium in the pyelocalyceal system (red arrow), Treatment: Laparoscopy. Ureterolysis. Section of the suture. JJ stent. Removal after 4 weeks

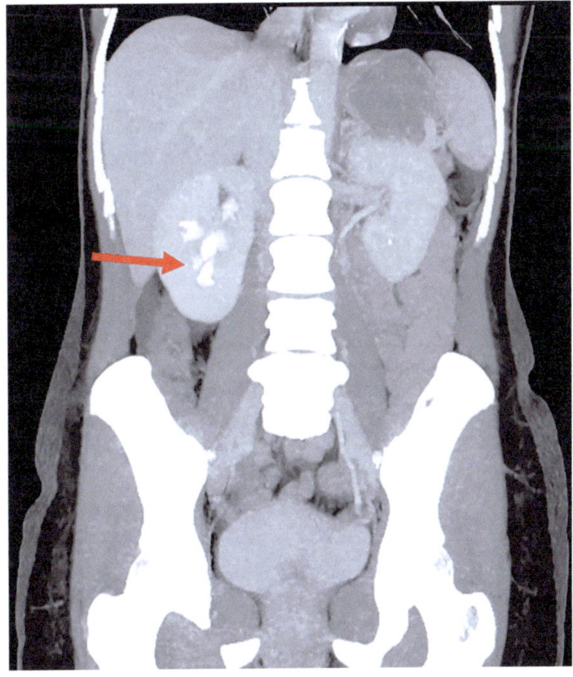

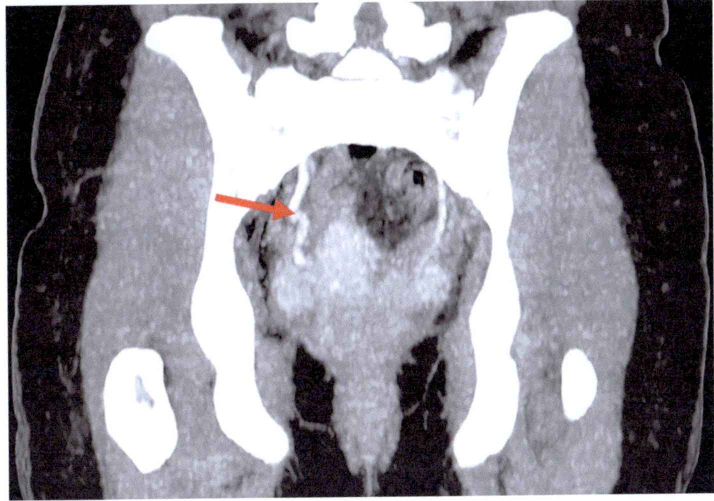

Fig. 9.3 Right ureteral kink. First postoperative day. CT-scan: coronal reconstruction with superposition of slices CT demonstrating the irregularity of the right distal ureter and dilatation in upper ureter (red arrow)

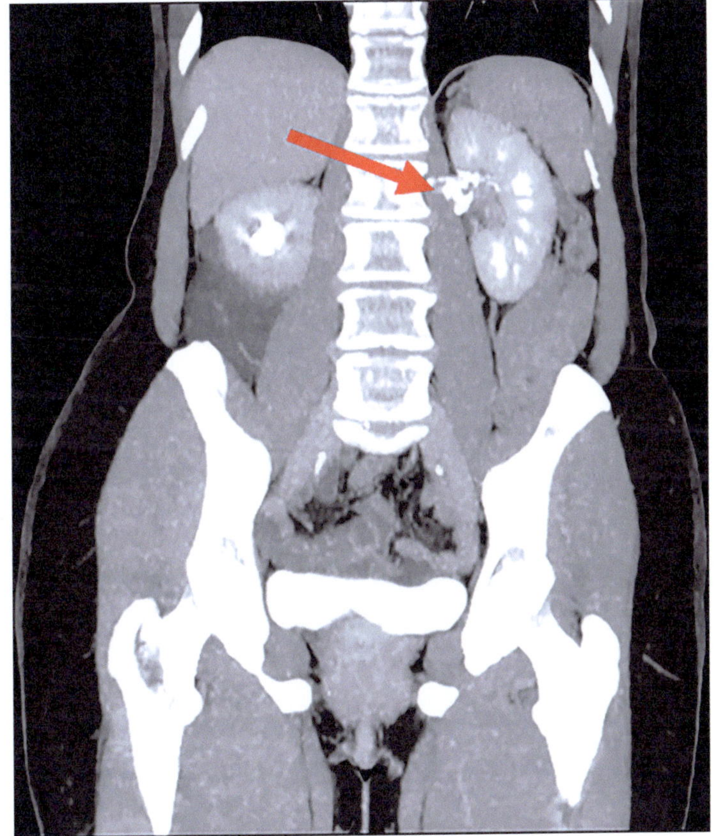

Fig. 9.4 Left pyelic rupture. Left ureteral obstruction by thermal injury following laparoscopic adnexectomy. Third postoperative day. CT-scan: Coronal reconstruction. Extravasation of contrast medium (red arrow). Treatment: Pigtail. Removal after 8 weeks. Stenosis. Reimplantation

Fig. 9.5 Postoperative left ureteral stenosis following. CT-scan. Ureteral dilatation above a distal ureteral stenosis of 2 cm (red arrow). The dilatation is sub-obstructive. There is no delay of excretion and the cortex of the kidney is respected

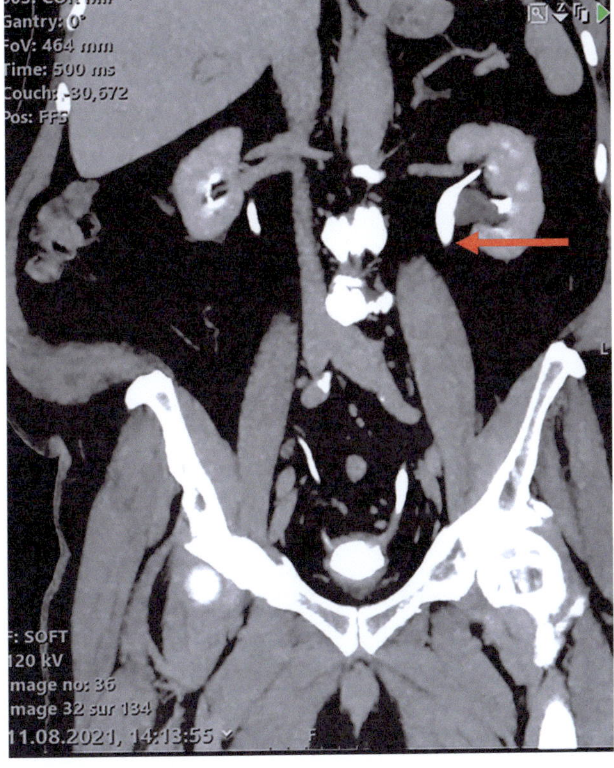

Fig. 9.6 Postoperative right ureteral stenosis, the same case, portal phasis. Preservation of the cortex of the kidney, confirming the absence of acute obstruction

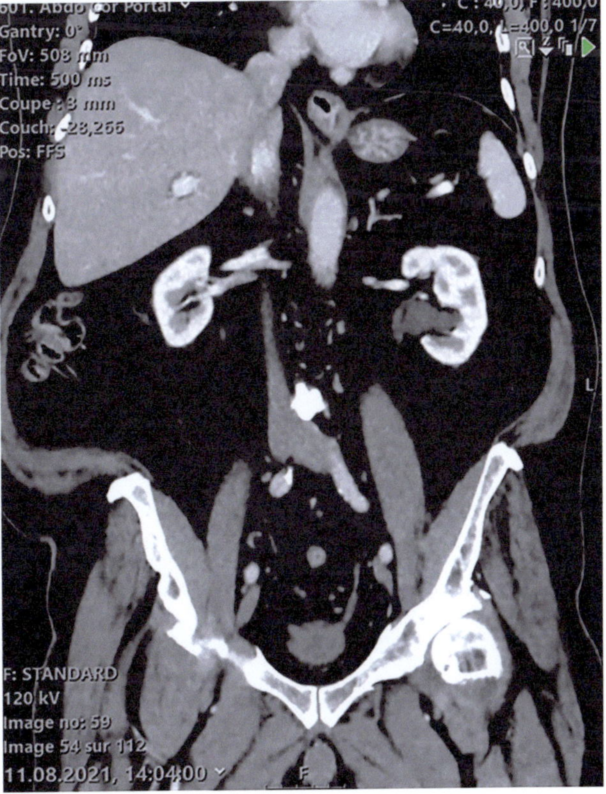

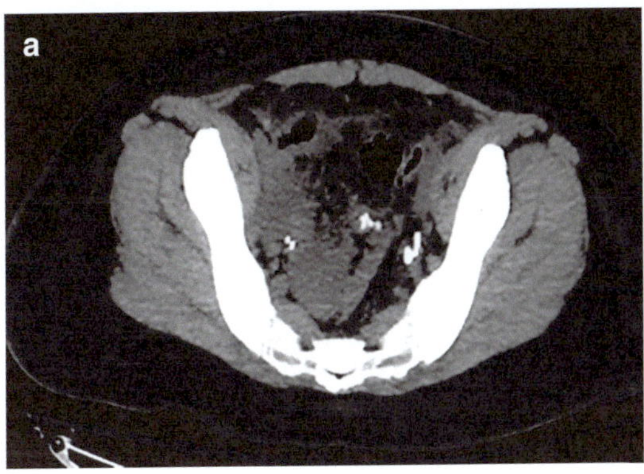

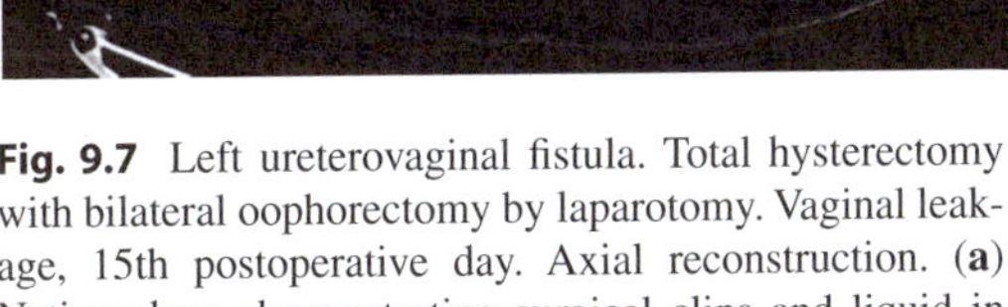

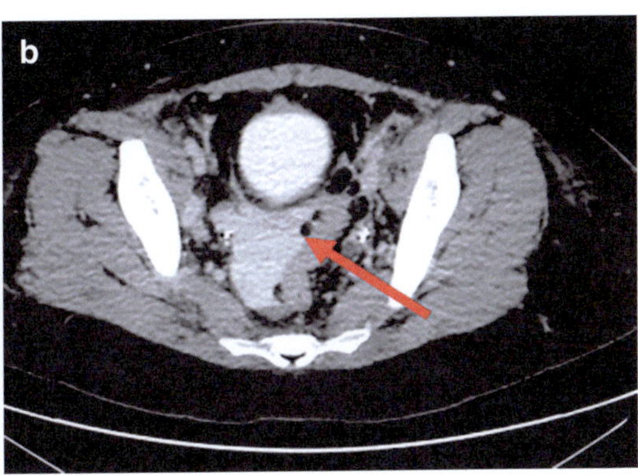

Fig. 9.7 Left ureterovaginal fistula. Total hysterectomy with bilateral oophorectomy by laparotomy. Vaginal leakage, 15th postoperative day. Axial reconstruction. (**a**) Native phase demonstrating surgical clips and liquid in Douglas. (**b**) With IV contrast in delayed phase demonstrating the extravasation of the contrast medium from the ureter (red arrow). Treatment: Percutaneous nephrostomy followed by reimplantation

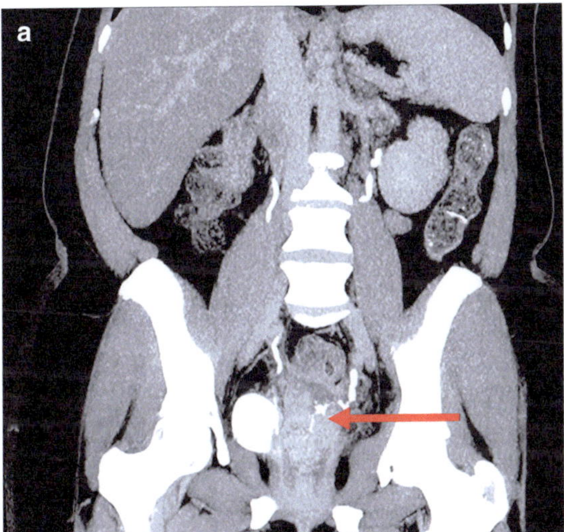

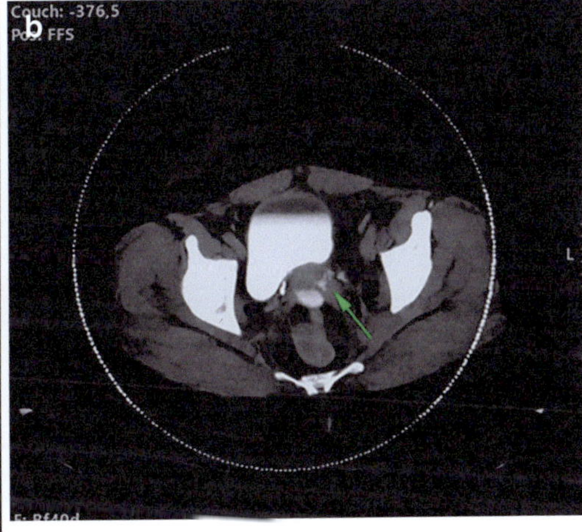

Fig. 9.8 Left ureterovaginal fistula. Thermal injury during difficult laparoscopic hysterectomy, 16th postoperative day. (**a**) CT-scan coronal reconstruction in a delayed phase CT after contrast-enhanced 10 min. Both ureters in proximal part are symmetric structures with contrast opacification. In the distal part, the contour of the left ureter is irregular with extravasation of the contrast around the ureter and with a vaginal communication (red arrow). (**b**) CT-scan axial reconstruction. Visualization of a left uterovaginal fistula (green arrow). Treatment: Pigtail. Removal after 8 weeks. Stenosis. Reimplantation

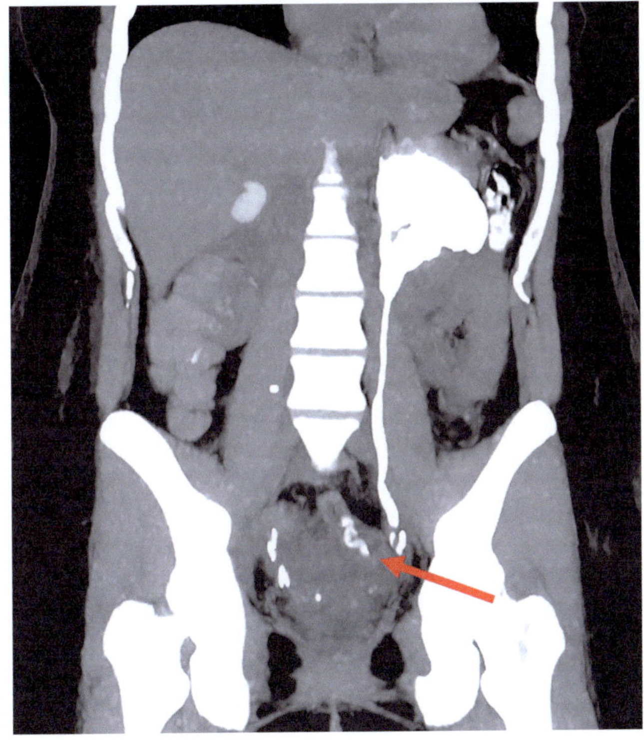

Fig. 9.9 Left ureterovaginal fistula. After total hysterectomy and adnexectomy by laparotomy. Ureterovaginal fistula (red arrow). 15th postoperative day. Coronal reconstruction. Contrast-enhanced perirenal (nephrostomy). Treatment: Percutaneous nephrostomy. Reimplantation

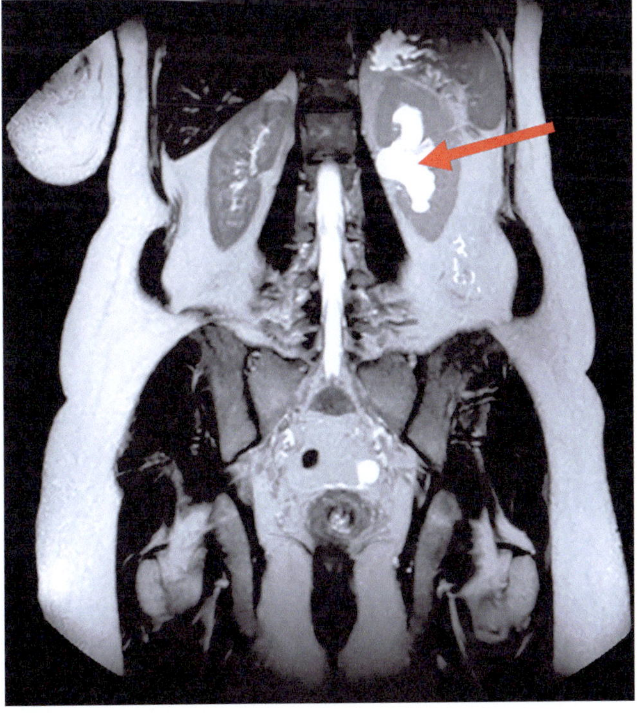

Fig. 9.10 Pelvic endometriotic nodule in contact with the distal left ureter. Left pyelocalicial dilatation (red arrow)

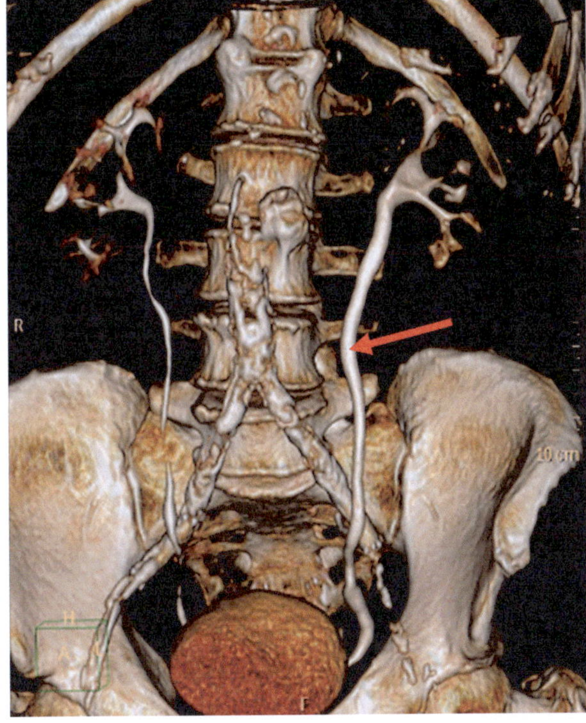

Fig. 9.11 Dilatation of the left ureter over its entire length. 3D CT-scan reconstruction demonstrating the asymmetry of the ureter diameters. Left ureter dilated (red arrow)

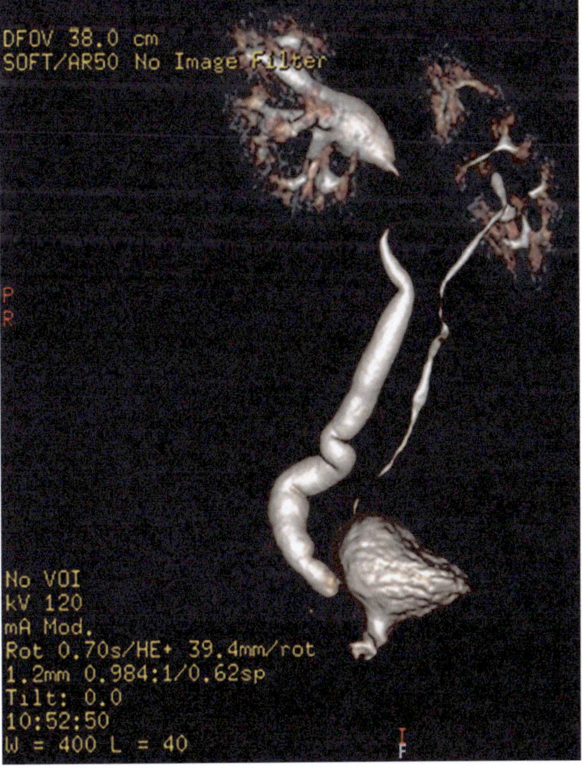

Fig. 9.12 Right distal obstruction of the ureter. Right pyelocalyceal and ureteral dilatation. 3D CT-scan reconstruction demonstrating the asymmetry of the ureter diameters

Fig. 9.13 Left distal obstruction. 3D reconstruction of a left distal obstruction (red arrow)

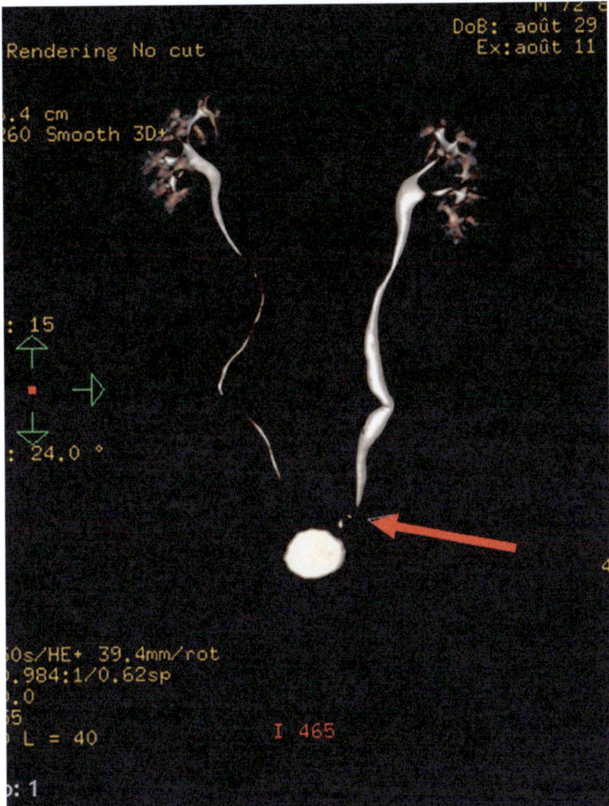

### 9.2.9	Intravenous Indocyanine Green Administration
(Figs. 9.14, 9.15, and 9.16)

Indocyanine green (ICG) is a fluorescent dye visible under near-infrared fluorescence (NIRF) light.

After intravenous administration (e.g., 5 ml of a 1% solution), well-vascularized tissue will rapidly show green fluorescence, differentiating it from ischemic or necrotic structures. This can be of value when assessing the vitality of the ureter when suspecting tissue damage or reconstructive surgery of the urinary tract.

Alternatively, it can be injected into the urinary tract (e.g., as a 0.25% solution), for example, to facilitate the anatomical identification of ureters during laparoscopy.

Fig. 9.14 Perioperative laparoscopic view. Bladder and distal left ureter following the complete resection of the endometriotic nodule. Ureteral "shaving" (red arrow). Left ureteral stent inserted before the procedure

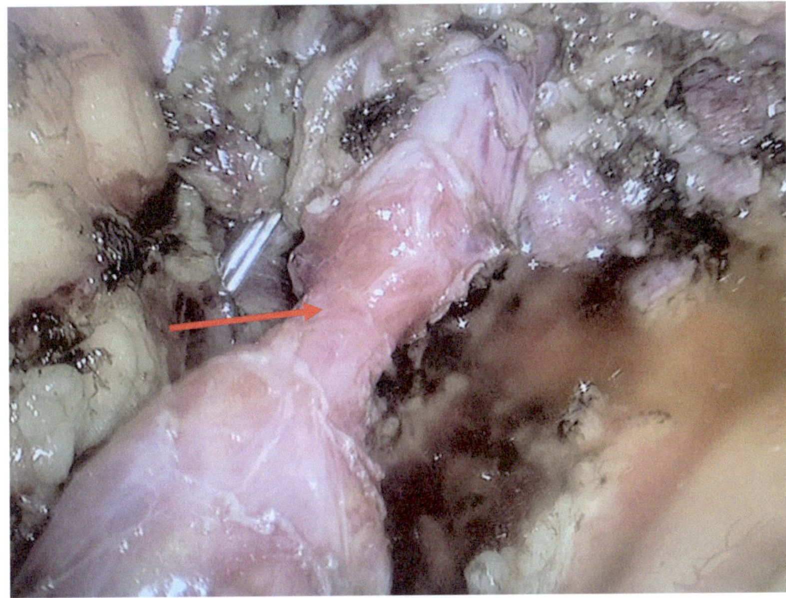

Fig. 9.15 Intravenous indocyanine green administration. For assessment of the vitality of the ureter. (1) Ureter, (2) Shaving area, correct vascularization

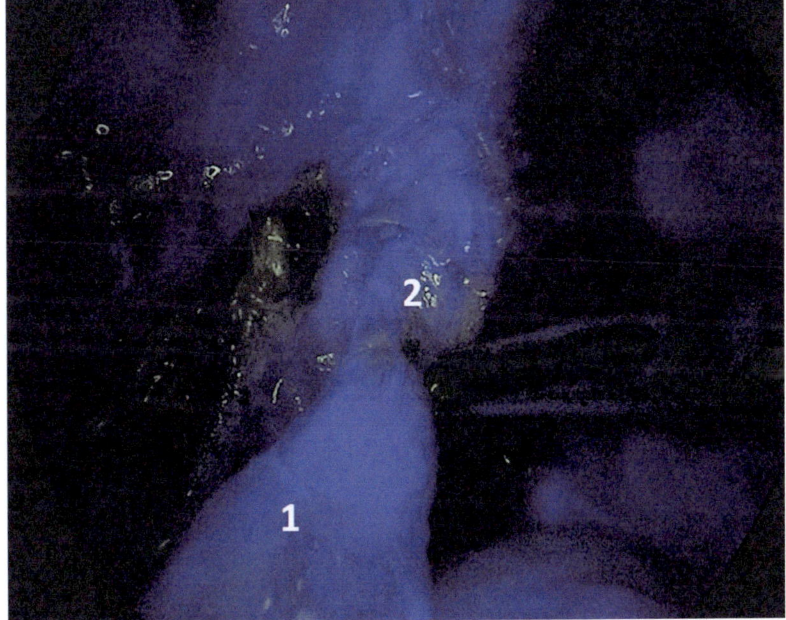

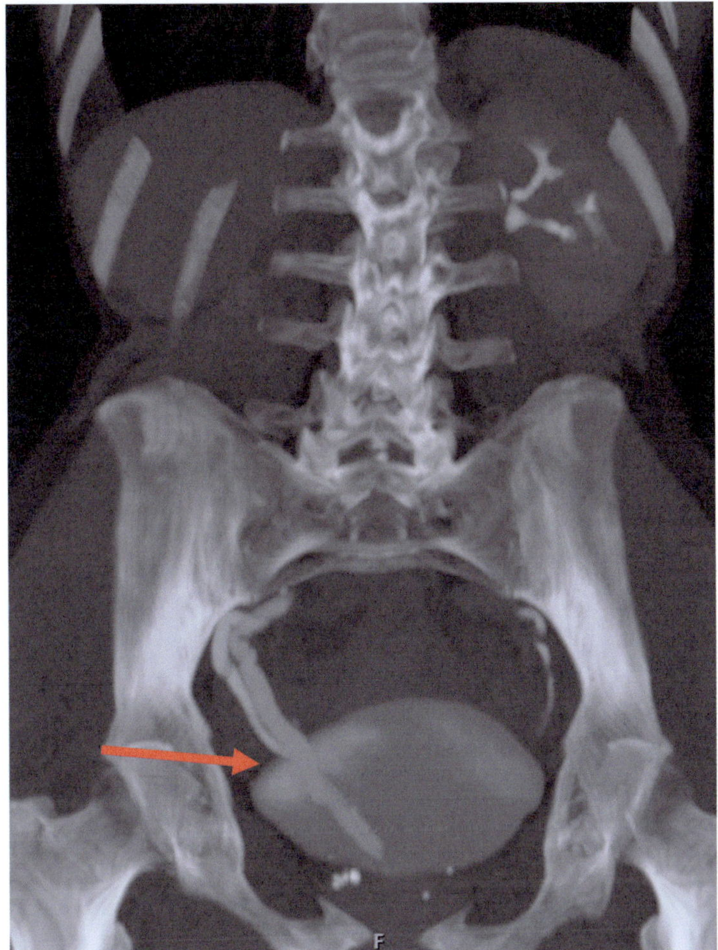

Fig. 9.16 Right duplex kidney with duplicated collecting system. Red arrow: visualisation of two ureteral sites of implantation at the level of the vesicoureteral junction

Treatment of the Ureteral Lesion

Chapter 10 concerns the treatments of the iatrogenic ureteral lesion during operation or the postoperative course. As soon as the ureteral injury is identified, immediate treatment is needed. Different drainage techniques are usually employed on an emergency basis, while the more complex reconstruction is performed once acute tissue damage has resolved.

10.1 Techniques for Urinary Drainage

Indications for drainage are on the one hand ureteral stenosis, which can be complicated by pain related to the distension of the collecting system, acute renal failure, obstructive pyelonephritis, and rupture of the renal pelvis due to distension; and on the other hand, urinary leakage. The subsequent urinoma may cause pain, induce fibrosis, compromise tissue regeneration, develop into a fistula, or become infected mostly with Gram-negative bacteria.

Three drainage techniques are commonly employed: endoscopic placement of a ureteral stent ("double-J catheter," "pigtail") or of a ureteral catheter ("single-J" catheter), or percutaneous placement of a nephrostomy tube.

Drainage achieves a definitive resolution of the injury in approximately half of the patients. In other words, it allows deferring final repair to a later stage under better surgical conditions.

10.1.1 Ureteral Stent (Double-J Catheter)

A ureteral stent drains urine from the renal pelvis into the bladder, its coiled ends hinder it from sliding out of the urinary tract. Several models are available with different lengths, widths, and degrees of rigidity. Generally, a large lumen will provide better drainage and is less at risk of obstruction by blood clots, pus, tissue debris, or other deposits. A rigid model is preferred in case of strong external compression, for example, in a long, tight, ischemic stricture. The stent should not be overly long and cross the bladder from side to side, as it is likely to cause more discomfort.

Stents are typically placed in a retrograde fashion under live fluoroscopy. A guidewire is pushed through the ureteral meatus up to the renal pelvis through a flexible or rigid cystoscope. The stent is then slid into position on the guidewire. This procedure can be performed in a variety of positions, depending on the degree of emergency, if the urethra is accessible in a sterile manner. A flexible cystoscope can reach the urethra in a supine position even if the legs are only minimally spread. Local anesthesia can be sufficient, but sedation, spinal or general anesthesia is preferred option if difficult stent placement is expected. In exceptional situations, placement can be performed without fluoroscopy. Renal ultrasound is then used to visualize the proximal coil in the renal pelvis.

If required, stents can be placed in an antegrade manner, i.e., through percutaneous renal access (see below) or during laparotomy/laparoscopy when performing immediate ureteral repair. In the latter case, intraoperative imaging is not required.

While a stent is the least invasive drainage method, its fully intracorporal position entails several drawbacks: diuresis from the drained kidney cannot be precisely measured, and neither can the quality of the urine be assessed (presence of pus, blood). Low-pressure drainage can only be obtained in association with a bladder catheter. If a stent obstruction is suspected, ultrasound or retrograde cystography must be performed, and a renewed procedure is required to change an obstructed stent.

However, a ureteral stent does not require specific care. Patients might experience urinary frequency and urgency, as well as lower abdominal and perineal pain while voiding, not unlike symptoms of a urinary tract infection. These usually lessen over time and can be managed with pain relief and spasmolytic medication (e.g., anticholinergic or beta-3-mimetic drugs). Sufficient hydration and diuresis will keep the stent permeable. A stent can be left in place for several months if need be.

10.1.2 Ureteral Catheter ("Single-J" Catheter)

Its placement is like that of a ureteral stent, but it has to be fixed to a Foley catheter. As it can be accessed from outside, exact urine output can be measured, and the catheter can be rinsed in case of significant hematuria or pyuria. Once these have resolved and diuresis is stable, it can be replaced by a double-J stent under fluoroscopy. In most cases, anesthesia is not necessary. A ureteral catheter requires careful nursing and is at risk of accidental dislocation.

10.1.3 Nephrostomy Tube

The nephrostomy tube is placed percutaneously under live fluoroscopy with or without additional ultrasound guidance. The patient is positioned in a flank or prone position. If needed, access can also be obtained if a supine patient is slightly turned sideways. The more the collecting system is distended, the easier is the tube placement. If there is no distension at all and retrograde stent placement is not possible, a puncture of the renal collecting system can be attempted under computer tomographic guidance.

Local anesthesia is usually sufficient, but in some cases, spinal or general anesthesia or sedation is preferred.

A nephrostomy tube is usually indicated when retrograde drainage fails or is not feasible, i.e., when the continuity of the ureter is lost due to a complete section of the ureter or its complete obstruction. It is therefore a useful reserve tool.

The main drawback of a nephrostomy tube is that the ureter is not aligned and held open. The regeneration of a ureteral injury may therefore be compromised. In most cases, a secondary procedure on the ureter will be necessary, ranging from antegrade stent placement to full surgical reconstruction of the ureter.

10.1.4 Success Rates of Ureteral Drainage

In the case of stenosis, stenting is more often successful if it is attempted early on, and if the ureteral obstruction is partial and limited in length. Simply placing a stent can resolve the problem in more than half of the cases. The stent is left for several weeks.

Morrow et al. [1] carried out, postoperatively, immediate treatment by the placement of a ureteral stent. Successful stenting was obtained in 11/21 (52%) with a median time to stent placement of 25 days (IQR 18.5–42). Those with failed stenting had a median time to attempted stenting of 65 days (IQR 10–91.3). Of those with successful stenting 3/11 (27%) had resolution requiring no further intervention. Open reconstruction was required in 6/11 (55%). These results confirm the interest in attempting to rise a ureteral catheter even in the postoperative late period.

In the management of late-diagnosed iatrogenic ureteral injuries, Lask et al. [2] published a study including 44 patients of whom 24 were treated primarily by immediate reconstructive surgery from 1979 to 1984 and 20 were treated primarily by percutaneous nephrostomy tube insertion beginning in 1985. The primary management of ureteral injury by percutaneous nephrostomy resulted in significantly decreased reoperation and morbidity rates and enabled spontaneous recovery of the injured ureter in most patients.

In the case of a ureterovaginal fistula and a minor ureteral lesion, ureteral stenting may be attempted as a sole treatment modality. Treatment failure will require surgical reconstruction.

10.2 Surgical Reconstruction

10.2.1 Ureteral Resection and Anastomosis (Ureteroureterostomy)

Direct ureteroureterostomy is the preferred option in injuries of the mid ureter (above the iliac vessels) that are up to 3 cm long and that cannot be mended by bladder reimplantation. More than ever, general principles of reconstructive surgery apply to this procedure: maintaining optimal blood supply through careful, thermal, and atraumatic dissection; and achieving a tension-free reconstruction through mobilization of the ureter. If both principles cannot be reconciled, an alternative method should be preferred. The same applies if tissue regeneration is compromised due to systemic or local conditions: cachexia, diabetes, chemotherapy, previous radiation therapy, local infection, urinoma, and endometriosis.

Depending on the setting, ureteroureterostomy is performed on the spot (i.e., directly when the ureter has been injured) or as a delayed procedure when conservative measures such as stent placement have failed.

Access is obtained by laparotomy or laparoscopy. Robotic assistance can facilitate tissue handling and suturing.

Ideally, the peritoneum is opened in such a way that it can be placed above the anastomosis once the procedure is finished. The ureter should be dissected with an intact adventitia. If present, periureteral vessels should be preserved. A vessel loop will provide atraumatic traction. The damaged ureteral segment is resected [3]. The ureteral ends should show some degree of bleeding, which will be controlled by the anastomotic suture. If in doubt, the vascularization of the ureteral ends can be assessed with ICG fluoroscopy. The tension of the resulting ends needs to be critically evaluated with the patient in a neutral position on the operating table. The ureters are then spatulated 1.5–2 cm on both ends and closed on a ureteral stent with thin (4/0–6/0) resorbable material. Both braided or monofilament, interrupted or running sutures can be used. Atraumatic handling of the ureters is paramount, for example, by using stay sutures and vessel loops.

Epiploic wrapping is indicated in the absence of peritoneum if the anastomosis needs to be isolated from surrounding tissues.

The Foley catheter is removed between postoperative days 5–10, and the stent after 2–6 weeks.

Paick et al. [4] observed good results by treating distal lesions even close to the bladder by anastomosis procedure. In their recent retrospective study, nine patients were successfully treated by resection and then anastomosis of the pelvic ureter with a 3-year follow-up. The lesion was distal, the length of the resected segment was 2.7 cm, and the distance from the section of the distal segment to the bladder junction was only 2.9 cm. Generally, however, the distal lesion is treated by reimplantation.

10.2.2 Ureterovesical Reimplantation (Ureteroneocystostomy)
(Figs. 10.1, 10.2, 10.3, 10.4, 10.5, 10.6, 10.7 and 10.8)

Ureteroneocystostomy is the method of choice to repair injuries of the distal third of the ureter, i.e., its iliac and pelvic sections. Located deep in the pelvis, the exposition and dissection of the distal segment are challenging and associated with a significant risk of secondary ischemia, stenosis, and leakage. The bladder, however, provides a malleable, well-vascularized, easily accessible landing zone for the proximal ureteral stump, even in case of major loss of length. Preoperative, retrograde cystography allows for visualizing bladder capacity, how high the bladder reaches cranially, and (if performed during retrograde ureterography) its anatomical relationship with the intact proximal ureter. Cystography is of relevance in heavily pretreated or operated patients in whom a loss of tissue elasticity or adherences are to be expected.

Generally, the iliac vessels are a useful landmark structure, as a healthy bladder can readily be mobilized to this level without additional tissue interposition.

The available length of the ureter and tissue quality impact must be considered when evaluating an antireflux mechanism. Prior to elective surgery, the reimplantation technique and its impact on bladder capacity must be discussed with the patient.

Reimplantation can be performed through open access (midline laparotomy or Pfannenstiel incision), as well as laparoscopically with or without robotic assistance, which is safe and effective. A sterile Foley catheter must be accessible to distend the bladder with saline solution to help mobilize and assess the waterproofness of the reconstruction. Depending on the situation, an extraperitoneal approach may be chosen.

There are three ways to gain additional length for ureteral reimplantation: bladder mobilization, psoas-hitch, and Boari-flap repair.

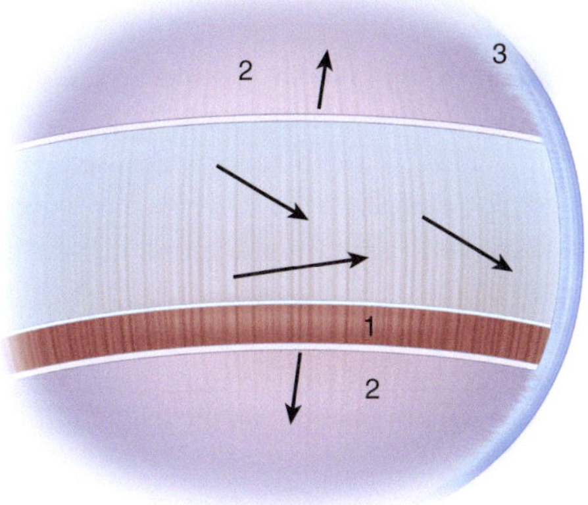

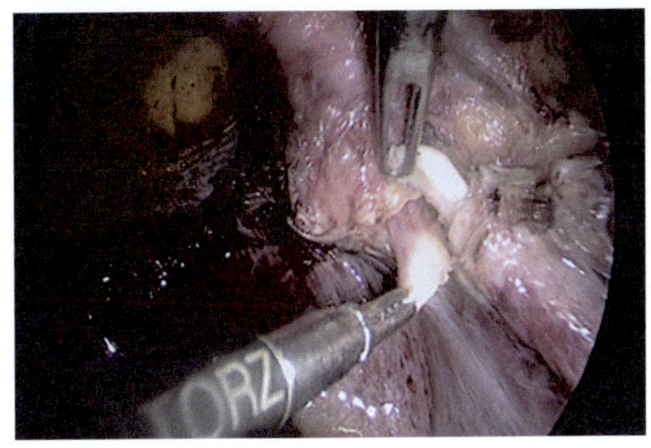

Fig. 10.1 Technique of uretero-vesical reimplantation with antireflux path. First step. Exposition of the bladder. Right side. Bladder visualization, incision of the peritoneum with the dissection of the Retzius space and then bladder mobilization. (1) Bladder, (2) peritoneum, (3) round ligament. Resection and repermeabilization of the ureter. Visualization and preparation of the two stumps before anastomosis (right side)

Fig. 10.2 Technique of uretero-vesical reimplantation with antireflux path. First step. Fixation of the bladder. Right side. After dissection of the Retzius space, mobilization of the bladder and attachment to the psoas muscle with few sutures. (1) Bladder, (2) peritoneum, (3) attachment to the psoas muscle

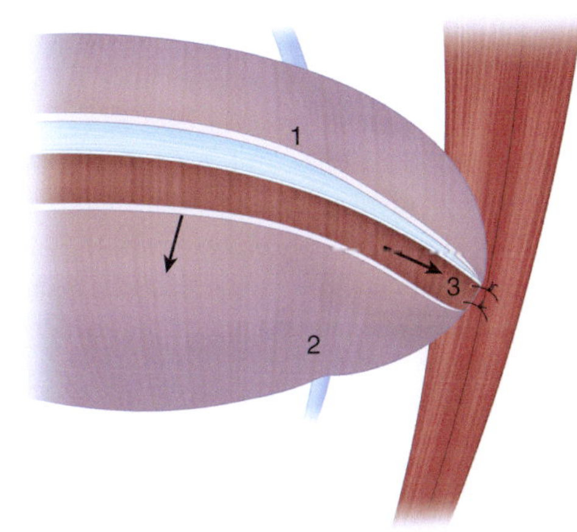

Fig. 10.3 Technique of uretero-vesical reimplantation with antireflux path. Second step. Preparation of the ureter. Section, mobilization of the ureter, no tension. Spatulation of the extremities of the ureter. With a short longitudinal incision of the end of the ureter. JJ Stent

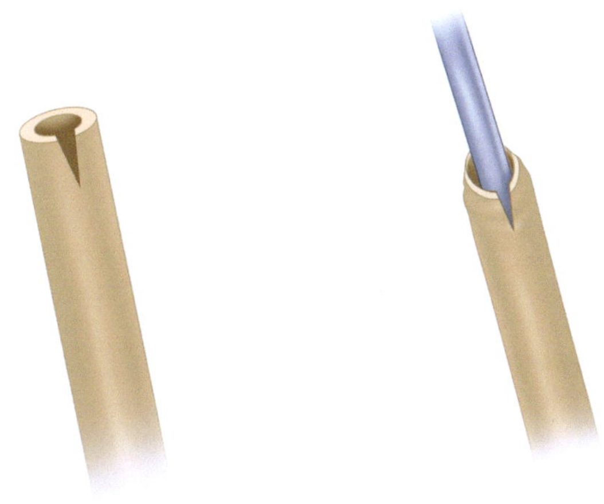

10.2.2.1 Bladder Mobilization

After dissecting the affected ureter, the whole anterior aspect of the bladder and the bladder dome are dissected. Filling the bladder with saline is helpful. The peritoneal tissue surrounding the ureter and bladder should be incised in such a way as to cover the resulting anastomosis. To help pull the bladder toward the affected ureter, its contralateral side is freed of its attachments, thereby sectioning its superior vascular pedicle and the umbilical artery. If needed, the dissection can be prolonged downward and include its inferior pedicle. Hemostasis is key. Normal anatomical planes are likely lost due to scarring, in particular after extensive debridement, infection, urine leakage, or radiation, but also unrelated procedures such as iliac vessel prosthesis. As the initial ureteral injury most likely happened for a reason, it is more than ever crucial to localize critical adjacent structures such as the external and internal iliac vein and artery, the obturator nerve (in case of extensive bladder mobilization), and the genitofemoral nerve (in particular during psoas-hitch). The proximal stump of the ureter must be handled with a stay suture and its adventitia kept intact as much as possible. The distal stump, if needed, is ligated or clipped.

If the mobilization of the bladder does not yield enough length, its anterior wall can be incised transversally and closed longitudinally in the intended direction (after the ureter has been reimplanted), in the manner of a pyloromyotomy. This will usually be combined with a fixation of the bladder dome to the psoas muscle. Before proceeding with opening the bladder, however, one must have decided whether or not to use a Boari-flap, as this requires specific tailoring of the detrusor.

10.2.2.2 Psoas-Hitch Technique

Once the bladder has been sufficiently mobilized and its anterior face incised, the postero-lateral aspect of its dome is sutured onto the psoas. This is achieved by separately placing three large, single stitches of slowly resorbable braided material (e.g., absorbable threads polyglactin 910, Vicryl 2/0®) into the thick of the detrusor muscle and the tendon of the psoas minor, or the muscle itself. The sutures are not tied until the resulting position of the bladder and their relationships to the ureteral stump have been verified. Mobilization of the bladder is facilitated by placing a few fingers in the transverse incision of the bladder wall. The genitofemoral nerve must not be taken into the sutures. The result should allow tension-free reimplantation. If that is not the case, and the bladder has already been maximally mobilized, a Boari-flap yields additional length.

10.2.2.3 Boari-Küss Flap Repair

If it is unlikely that the fully mobilized bladder will reach the ureter, in particular, if it is sectioned several centimeters above the iliac artery, a broad bladder flap is rotated upward, anastomosed onto the ureter, and closed in a cylindrical manner.

On the dome and anterior aspect of the fully distended bladder, electric cautery is used to mark the intended flap. Its tip is situated on the lower part of the contralateral anterior bladder wall. The outline of the flap must have the shape of a broad arch, in particular in a situation of poor vascularization. As a rule of thumb, the flap's base should measure no less than a third of its length. The flap is then tilted diagonally upward across the iliac vessels and anchored on the psoas with two or three 3/0 resorbable stitches. Once the ureter has been reimplanted and stented, the bladder is closed with a longitudinal suture.

10.2.2.4 Anastomosis Technique

The single overbearing goal is to achieve a well-vascularized, tension-free anastomosis with a well-spatulated ureter. An antireflux mechanism will require additional ureteral length and should only be employed without compromising these principles. In poorly vascularized tissue, for example, in patients after radiation, chemotherapy, or major systemic diseases, less is more.

The proximal ureter is sectioned above its injured part and fitted with a stay suture. Correct vascularization is assessed visually. ICG-fluorescence provides an elegant addition. The ureteral stump is then spatulated over 1–2 cm and brought to its landing site on the bladder.

Fig. 10.4 Technique of uretero-vesical reimplantation with antireflux path. Third step. Incision of the detrusor. Right side. 3 cm incision of the detrusor without opening of the mucosa. (1) Incision of the detrusor, (2) intact mucosa, (3) attached bladder to the psoas muscle

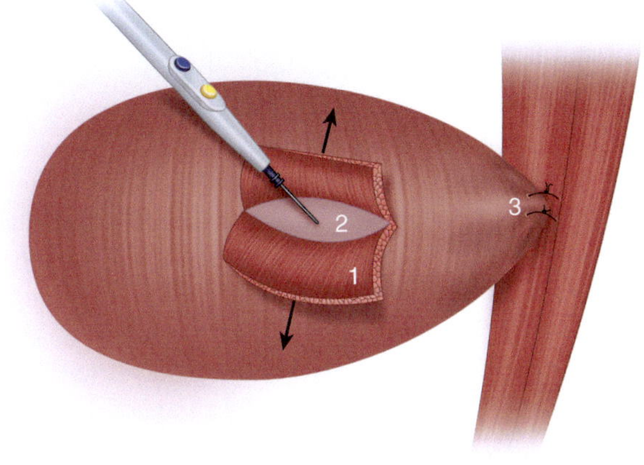

Fig. 10.5 Technique of uretero-vesical reimplantation with antireflux path. Forth step. Incision of the mucosa and ureteral approximation. Short incision of the mucosa with a monopolar needle. (1) Detrusor, (2) Incision of the mucosa

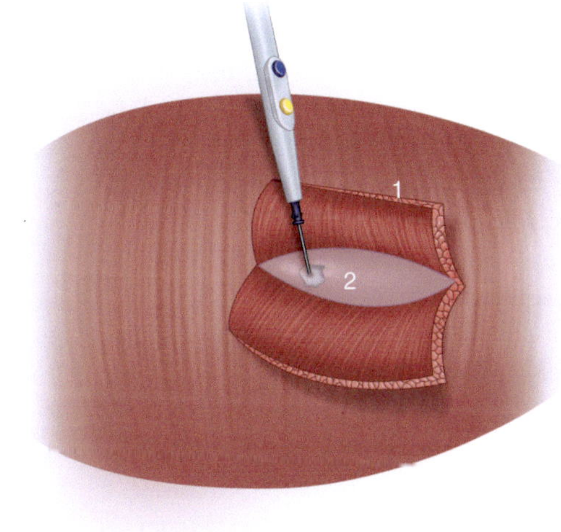

For a simple, refluxing anastomosis, the bladder wall is incised to create a direct and short passage for the ureter, which is brought in place by pulling on its stay suture. Ureterovesical anastomosis is then done mucosa to mucosa with thin (4/0–6/0) sutures, either with interrupted or running sutures. Stitches include the mucosa and submucosal tissue. The proximal angle of the spatulated ureter should not be tightened by the sutures. Rather, they should spread this angle wide open. Monofilament material is less likely to tear the thin ureteral tissue. Additional sutures can be placed on the serosa and the anastomosis is covered with peritoneum.

An antireflux mechanism is commonly performed according to Lich-Gregoir [5, 6]. It is attained by passing the distal centimeter of the ureter through a submucosal tunnel. The bladder is filled with saline and its serosa and detrusor muscle incised 3 cm on the intended landing site. On the medial end of the incision, the bladder mucosa is opened over a few millimeters and the ureter is pulled into the bladder lumen, where its spatulated end is sutured mucosa to mucosa as above. Then, the detrusor is closed over the ureter without compressing it using separate absorbable 3/0 or 2/0 stitches.

The Boari technique with a tubular bladder flap is rarely required in gynecology. Its success rate is over 95%, whether done openly or laparoscopically [7, 8], or with robotic assistance [9].

Regardless of the reimplantation technique, a ureteral stent is placed before the bladder is closed and kept for a minimum of 2 weeks. Its correct position should be checked with abdominal plain film radiography no later than postoperative day 1. A bladder catheter is kept in place between 2 and 7 days depending on the extension of the bladder suture. In cases with compromised tissue regeneration, a retrograde cystography can be used before catheter removal, as it will reveal leaks requiring prolonged catheterization. The bladder must be adequately distended, i.e., nearly up to its functional capacity. Post-drainage or oblique X rays are required to visualize anterior and posterior leaks. Reflux along the ureteral stent is commonly observed.

Once the bladder catheter has been removed, transient discomfort related to the stent and the bladder suture is to be expected. The patient must be informed of this beforehand. Medication can alleviate symptoms (ref. Sect. 10.1.1).

10.2.2.5 Additional Ureteral Repair Techniques

In exceptional cases, additional techniques can be of help. The kidney can be dissected from the Gerota fascia and mobilized downward with the proximal ureter. In ureterotransureterostomy, a shortened, injured ureter is pulled through the mesocolon above the inferior mesenteric artery and anastomosed on the contralateral ureter. Buccal mucosa grafts can be used for ureteroplasty on any part of the proximal and iliac ureter. For long ureteral injuries, ileal or appendicular interposition segments can be useful. These rarely employed methods are described in specialized articles and are beyond the scope of this book.

Fig. 10.6 Technique of uretero-vesical reeimplantation with antireflux path. Forth step. Approximation. Approximation of the ureteral extremity to the vesical mucosa (JJ stent). (1) Ureter, (2) JJ stent

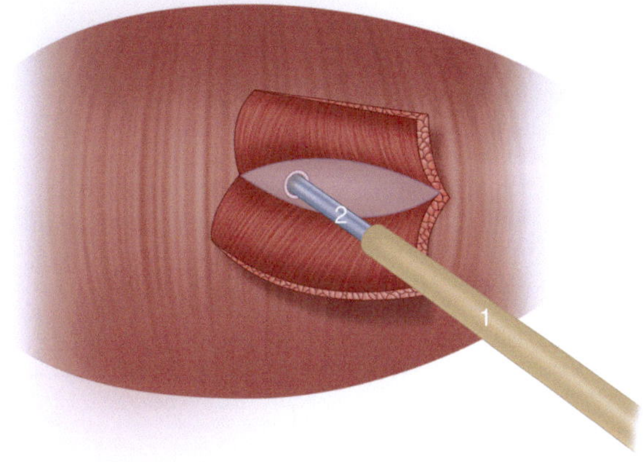

Fig. 10.7 Technique of uretero-vesical reeimplantation with antireflux path. Fifth step. Reimplantation with suture. (1) Separate sutures bladder mucosa-ureter

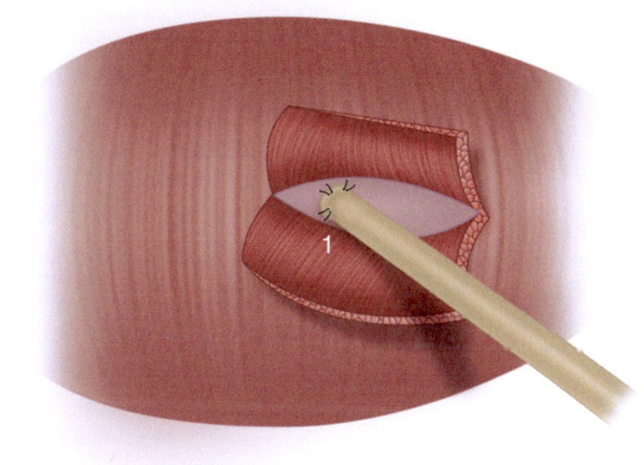

Fig. 10.8 Technique of uretero-vesical reimplantation with antireflux path. Sixth step. Closure of the detrusor (tunnelization). With few sutures. (1) Detrusor, (2) ureter

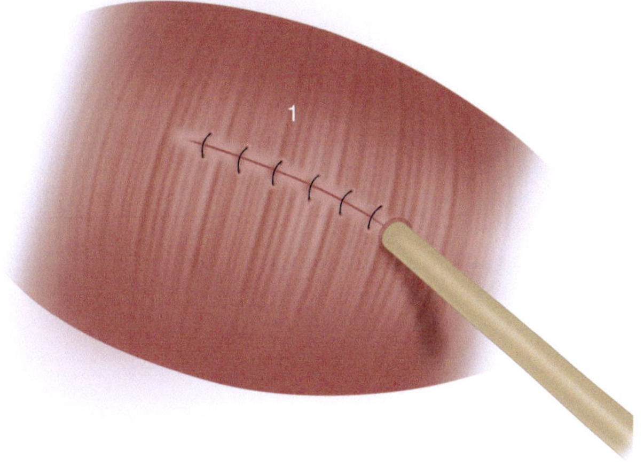

References

1. Morrow J, Curry D, Dooher M, Woolsey S. Minimally invasive management of delayed recognition iatrogenic ureteric injury. Ulster Med J. 2017;86(3):181–4.
2. Lask D, Abarbanel J, Luttwak Z, Manes A, Mukamel E. Changing trends in the management of iatrogenic ureteral injuries. J Urol. 1995;154(5):1693–5.
3. Smith I, Cooper M. Management of ureteric endometriosis associated with hydronephrosis: an Australian case series of 13 patients. BMC Res Notes. 2010;3:45.
4. Paick JS, Hong SK, Park MS, Kim SW. Management of postoperatively detected iatrogenic lower ureteral injury: should ureteroureterostomy really be abandoned? Urology. 2006;67(2):237–41.
5. Lich R. Recurrent urosepsis in children. J Urol. 1961;86:554–8.
6. Gregoir W. Le reflux vesicourétéral congénital. Urol Int. 1962;30:286–300.
7. Rassweiller JJ, Gozen AS, Erdogru T, Sugiono M, Teber T. Ureteral Reimplantation for Management of Ureteral Strictures: a retrospective comparison of laparoscopic and open techniques. Eur Urol. 2007;51(2):512–22.
8. Gosen AG, Cresswell J, Canda AE, Ganta S, Rassweiler J, Teber D. Laparoscopic ureteral Reimplantation: prospective evaluation of medium-term results and current developments. World J Urol. 2010;28(2):221–6.
9. Stolzenburg JU, Rai BP, Do M, Dietel A, Liasikos E, Granzer R, Quazi H, Meneses AD, Lallidonis H. Robot-assisted technique for Boari flap ureteric reimplantation: replicating the techniques of open surgery in robotics. BJU Int. 2016;118(3):482–4.

Part IV

Ureteral Endometriosis

Ureteral Endometriosis

11

J.-B. Dubuisson et al., *Ureteral Complications of Gynecological Surgery*,
https://doi.org/10.1007/978-3-031-15598-7_11

Chapter 11 is devoted to ureteral endometriosis. It includes definitions of extrinsic and intrinsic ureteral endometriosis and procedures used for diagnosis. The different treatments are described and discussed including the excision of endometriotic lesions, ureterolysis, segmental resection/ureteral reimplantation, and medical treatments.

11.1 Frequency of Ureteral Endometriosis

The main condition affecting the pelvic ureter in women is endometriosis. Ureteral endometriosis is rare, less than 1% of endometriosis cases [1, 2]. Palla et al. [3] estimate that the ureter is the second most frequent site of urinary endometriosis after the bladder, followed by the ureter, kidney, and urethra with rates of 40%, 5%, 1%, and 1%.

11.2 Definitions

Extrinsic ureteral endometriosis is distinguished from intrinsic endometriosis. Either extrinsic or intrinsic endometriosis may result in partial or total obstruction and finally ureterohydronephrosis.

11.2.1 Extrinsic Endometriosis

Extrinsic endometriosis is four times more common. It concerns all lesions that include the ureter, such as the deep infiltrating nodule, extensive implants from the uterosacral ligament, stenosing fibrous adhesions, ovarian endometrioma as well as bladder endometriosis [4]. Ureteral endometriosis often involves the lower part of the pelvic ureter on a short segment in contact with the uterine artery, most often on the left.

11.2.2 Intrinsic Endometriosis

Intrinsic endometriosis affects the ureteral wall itself with the involvement of the muscularis or even the mucosa.

11.3 Diagnosis of Ureteral Endometriosis

The diagnosis of ureteral endometriosis may be suspected clinically and confirmed during a laparoscopy performed to evaluate chronic pelvic pain. It can also be diagnosed by imaging for the staging of pelvic endometriosis, especially deep infiltrating endometriosis. It is sometimes unknown and asymptomatic, discovered incidentally because of renal impairment or ureterohydronephrosis.

11.4 Treatments of Ureteral Endometriosis

The treatment indicated for ureteral endometriosis is surgical and always difficult. The surgical management is most often performed by laparoscopy. Medical treatments, mainly GnRh agonists, are prescribed in the event of an immediate contraindication to surgery and may be associated with the placement of a ureteral stent.

11.4.1 Excision of all Pelvic Endometriotic Lesions

In the first step, the excision of pelvic endometriotic lesions must be carried out. There are various procedures.

The resection of a nodule of the rectovaginal septum is often difficult and may need the collaboration of a visceral surgeon in case of a large rectal or sigmoid infiltration. The dissection of infiltrating intestinal placards is delicate with the risk of bowel injury. The presence of an adherent ovarian endometrioma obliges to be as conservative as possible in women with a desire to be pregnant because of the risk of ovarian reserve impairment.

A vesicovaginal or vesicouterine nodule may be associated with ureteral endometriosis. The preoperative assessment is mandatory for the precise extension of the lesions and the involvement of the urinary tract (cystoscopy, CT urography).

Rarely, do the vesicouterine lesions extend toward the trigone and involve the intravesical portion of the ureter. These vesicoureteral lesions are often complex and complicate surgical management.

Laparoscopic excision consists of removing as much of the pathological nodular or infiltrating tissue as possible. Then the ureter, whether it is included in the nodule or the infiltration, or whether it is inherently pathological itself, must be treated at the same time, especially if there is an overlying impact.

11.4.2 Ureterolysis

Ureterolysis is one of the procedures associated with the resection of endometriotic lesions close to the ureter. Ureterolysis is the first treatment performed, especially if ureteric pain is present. It can be followed by the placement of a ureteral catheter for several weeks. Many authors report the favorable results of ureterolysis [5].

Ghezzi et al. [1] report, that in a prospective multicenter cohort, 85% success in 33 women with a moderate or severe obstructive lesion of the ureter with a mean follow-up of 16 months.

In the Smith and Cooper series [6] of 13 patients with endometriosis associated with hydronephrosis, ureterolysis was sufficient in 7 of 13 cases (53.8%) without ureteral stenting, and in 3 cases (23.1%) associated with a JJ stent. Only 3 of 13 cases (23.1%) had to be treated with ureteral resection.

More recently, Knabben et al. [7] observed that 98.1% of cases of ureteral endometriosis were treated by ureterolysis. Even with an obstructive lesion, ureterolysis provided sufficient drainage from the kidney (86.7% of cases).

The publication by Cavaco-Gomes et al. goes in the same direction [8]. They analyzed 18 articles including 700 patients with ureteral endometriosis. 57% had at least one surgery for endometriosis. Ureterohydronephrosis was observed in 48.3% of patients. Most of the patients did not have specific urinary symptoms. Ureterolysis was sufficient in 86.7% of treatment cases. The remaining cases required ureteral

resection. Involvement of the rectovaginal septum and uterosacral ligaments was present in 58.8% and 47.9% of cases, respectively. Concomitant bladder endometriosis was noted in 18.8% of cases. During follow-up, only 3.9% of patients experienced persistence or recurrence of endometriosis.

Darwish et al. [9] observed equivalent results. Ureteral lesions were treated by ureterolysis in 78% of the patients and by primary segmental resection in 22%. No patient required nephrectomy. Histological analysis revealed intrinsic ureteral endometriosis in 54.5% of cases.

11.4.3 Segmental Resection

Segmental resection is sometimes necessary for extensive or stenosing parietal involvement since ureterolysis is sometimes ineffective in treating ureteral dilation.

The first publications on the laparoscopic treatment of posterior deep infiltrating lesions of endometriosis, including that of Nezhat et al. [10], had shown that ureterolysis was not always sufficient and that resection-anastomosis or ureterocystoneostomy was sometimes necessary. Other authors also weighed the effectiveness of simple ureterolysis in several cases [3, 11].

Mereu et al. [2] report a prospective series of 56 patients with moderate or severe ureteral dilation. Of the 35 cases treated by laparoscopic ureterolysis, 11 (31.4%) presented major complications while of the 17 cases treated by ureteroureterostomy only 2 (11.7%) had complications.

Miranda-Mendoza et al. [12] retrospectively report 13 cases of severe deep endometriosis associated with severe ureterohydronephrosis. All were treated by resection of pelvic endometriotic lesions by laparoscopy. Ureterolysis was possible in 53.8% of cases, but this had to be completed by end-to-end resection and anastomosis in 46.2% of the other cases. Severe postoperative complications were noted in three cases.

Alves et al. [5] reported that among 658 cases of deep infiltrating posterior endometriosis, 198 ureteral involvement required ureterolysis. Among these 198 cases, 28 were severe with ureteral dilation and hydronephrosis. Among these 28 cases, we note 15 ureterolysis, 12 anastomosis, 1 reimplantation within the aftermath 3 reoperations: 1 case of ureterovaginal fistula, 1 case of dilation with hydronephrosis, and 1 case of persistent pain.

11.4.4 Reimplantation

Reimplantation or ureteroneocystostomy is sometimes the only surgical option due to the extent of pelvic and ureteral lesions. Ceccaroni et al. [13] recently insisted on the interest of a broad indication of the technique of ureteroneocystostomy performed by laparoscopy. They report 160 cases of deep posterior endometriosis with ureteral involvement (intrinsic 45.6%, 54.4% extrinsic). All the cases were treated by endometriotic resection and ureteroneocystostomy with psoas bladder in 58.7% of cases. Bowel resection was necessary in 75.6% of cases. They only note a reoperation rate of 4.4%, intestinal fistula of 1.9%, and urination disorders of 15% after 6 months. Recurrence of endometriosis is noted in 1.2% of cases. Such results are very encouraging. It should be remembered that complementary medical treatment is often associated with surgical treatment in severe forms.

References

1. Ghezzi F, Cromi A, Bergamini V, Boils P. Management of ureteral endometriosis, areas of controversy. Curr Opin Obstet Gynecol. 2007 aug;19:319–24.
2. Mereu L, Gagliardi ML, Clarizia R, Mainardi P, Landi S, Minelli L. Laparoscopic management of ureteral endometriosis in case of moderate-severe hydroureteronephrosis. Fertil Steril. 2010 jan;93(1):46–51.
3. Palla VV, Karaolanis G, Katafigiotis I, Anastasiou I. Ureteral endometriosis: a systematic literature review. Indian J Urol. 2017;33(4):276–82.
4. Umar SA, MacLennan GT, Cheng L. Endometriosis of the ureter. J Urol. 2008;179:2412.
5. Alves J, Puga M, Fernandes R, Pinton A, Miranda I, Kovoor E, Wattiez A. Laparoscopic management of ureteral endometriosis and hydronephrosis associated with endometriosis. J Minim Invasive Gynecol. 2017;24(3):466–72.
6. Smith I, Cooper M. Management of ureteric endometriosis associated with hydronephrosis: an Australian case series of 13 patients. BMC Res notes. 2010;3:45.
7. Knabben L, Imboden S, Fellmann B, Nirgianakis K, Kuhn A, Mueller MD. Urinary tract endometriosis in patients with deep infiltrating endometriosis: prevalence, symptoms, management, and proposal for a new clinical classification. Fertil Steril. 2015;103:147–52.
8. Cavaco-Gomes J, Martinho M, Gilabert-aguilar J, Gilabert-estélles J. Laparoscopic management of ureteral endometriosis: a systematic review. Eur J Obstet Gynecol Reprod Biol. 2017 mar;210:94–101.
9. Darwish B, Stochino-Loi E, Pasquier G, Dugardin F, Defortescu G, Abo C, Roman H. Surgical outcomes of urinary tract deep infiltrating endometriosis. J Minim Invasive Gynecol. 2017 sep-oct;24(6):998–1006.
10. Nezhat C, Silfen S, Nezhat F, Martin D. Surgery for endometriosis. Curr Opin Obstet Gynecol. 1991 Jun;3(3):385–93.
11. Lich R. Recurrent urosepsis in children. J Urol. 1961;86:554–8.
12. Miranda-Mendoza I, Kovoor E, Nassif J, Ferreira H, Wattiez A. Laparoscopic surgery for severe ureteric endometriosis. Eur J Obstet Gynecol Reprod Biol. 2012 dec;165(2):275–9.
13. Ceccaroni M, Ceccarello M, Caleffi G, Clarizia R, Scarperi S, Pastorello M, Molinari A, Ruffo G, Cavalleri S. Total Laparoscopic ureteroneocystostomy for ureteral endometriosis: a single-center experience of 160 consecutive patients. J Minim Invasive Gynecol. 2019 jan;26(1):78–86.

Take Home Message

1. "You have to see the ureter and avoid it rather than avoid seeing it."
2. Total hysterectomy is the main operation responsible for ureteral injuries.
3. The areas where the ureter may be injured during gynecological procedures are (1) the crossing of the uterine artery, (2) the crossing of the iliac vessels, and (3) the distal insertion of the infundibulopelvic ligament.
4. Intraoperative checking of the integrity of both ureters is recommended during any pelvic operation with a risk of ureteral injury. It includes checking ureteral caliber and peristalsis, even if the presence of these clinical signs does not eliminate a ureteric injury.
5. Intraoperative cystoscopy with intravenous injection of indigo carmine is useful if a ureteral injury is suspected.
6. A normal cystoscopy does not eliminate a ureteral lesion, especially in case of thermal injury.
7. The discovery of a ureteral injury requires immediate treatment.
8. Complications related to missed ureteral injuries are often delayed in the postoperative period (till 2 or 3 weeks), especially for the formation of the ureter fistula.
9. In case of severe pelvic infiltrating endometriosis, management of ureteral endometriosis is mandatory because of the underlying renal risks. It must be accompanied by the excision of the surrounding endometriotic lesions to avoid a high risk of recurrence.